Disclaimer: Results may vary, and any testimonials are not claimed to represent typical results. All testimonials are real, and all the men and women pictured transformed their bodies using Jessica Kiernan's techniques. However, these results are meant as a showcase of what the best, most motivated clients have done and should not be taken as average or typical results. In addition, you assume certain risks inherent in exercise and nutrition programs by reading this book and viewing any related videos. The Fierce Abs workout program involves body weight exercises, weight lifting, and high intensity cardiovascular exercise. You should not begin the program if you are severely obese, or if you have a physical condition that makes intense exercise dangerous. In addition, the Fierce Abs program and/or Jessica Kiernan may suggest you follow an eating plan and at times restrict the amount of calories you consume. You should not begin this or any eating plan if you have physical or psychological issues which make fat loss dangerous. Jessica is not a doctor, and her advice is not a substitute for medical advice. Consult your physician before beginning any exercise or nutrition program. See our full Terms of Use and Privacy Policy for complete details @ www.JessicaKiernan.com.

FIERCE ABS: YOUR JUMP START GUIDE TO SCULPT, TIGHTEN & TONE YOUR ABS

All Rights Reserved.

Published by JK Media, LLC
Copyright © 2013 by JK Media, LLC
Cover art by Luis Escobar

This book is protected under the copyright laws of the United States of America. No part of this book may be reproduced or transmitted in any form or by any means, electronic or mechanical, including photocopying, recording, or by any information storage and retrieval system without the written permission of the author.

First Printing: January 2013
Printed in the United States of America.

First Edition: January 2013

# FIERCE ABS

## YOUR JUMP START GUIDE TO SCULPT, TIGHTEN & TONE YOUR ABS

Jessica Kiernan

Table of Contents

Introduction…..1
Free "Fierce Abs" Video Series…..3

Part 1
The Abdominal Muscles and Their Functions…..5
The Abs You Already Have…..9
A Look in the Mirror: Stand up for Yourself…..10
Understanding Your Body…..12

Part 2
Set Your Goals…..20
Building on Your Foundation…..32
Extra Fierce Exercises…..51
The Big HIIT…..58
Keeping it Flat by Not Working Flat…..64

Part 3
Keeping it Fresh…..66
The Best, the Good, the Bad and the Ugly…..70
The Must Have Grocery List…..110

Part 4
Just Say "Na"…..111
Bad Smoothie!…..114
Fat Burners?…..117
Relax Your Way to Fierce Abs…..120
Final Tips and Summary…..122
Questions or Comments?…..125

# Introduction

This book is dedicated to helping you achieve the fierce abdominal muscles you've always wanted. This muscle group, commonly called abs, six pack, washboard and other less common monikers, is one of the core muscle groups in your body.

The abdominal muscles are a group of 6 muscles that extend from your rib cage down to your pelvic bones. They allow you to move your trunk (chest, abdomen and back) in various ways; they also provide support for the trunk, often called the *core*. Additionally, they assist in the breathing process.

In this book you will start out with a self-assessment and then, based on that, begin setting your goals. Based on these two things we'll work together to develop a tailored exercise routine and diet plan to achieve fierce abs!

Your Fitness and Nutrition Coach... Hi, I'm Jess. "Fitness, nutrition, & motivation" is my slogan and it's what I live by! Growing up I ate terrible and didn't pay attention to what I put in my body. Because I had little guidance, it was up to me to change my habits and my lifestyle.

When I came across the Kiana Tom Fitness TV show I realized that I wanted to be healthy and that fitness and nutrition was something that I was very interested in. I wanted to look like that! But I also realized I needed a coach, I couldn't do it alone...

I started learning about nutrition, how to work out properly and proper form from a close friend and personal trainer and I began helping my friends and family get on the right track too. I have to admit I loved the excitement of helping, transforming, and motivating people.

A short time later I got certified and formally became a Personal Trainer. I am certified through AAAI/ISMA as a Phase I and II Master Trainer & a Nutritional Consultant. I am also constantly reading and learning and searching for new techniques and new information on fitness and nutrition to help my clients. I am always taking things to next level and going bigger and better and I challenge everyone to go further, go harder, and keep making goals!

I have been passionate about health and fitness for over 10 years and I will help you learn to make healthier lifestyle choices, lose pounds, and improve your endurance and strength! I will help motivate and inspire you to become the best YOU can be.

I recently launched www.JessicaKiernan.com a blog and informational site to help the world get fit and stay healthy where I offer various products and services to all of my clients and fans. Check it out!

My most rewarding project is www.FierceMinute.com which is a FREE video training program to help folks each day with a fitness or nutrition tip. It's fun and straight-forward and the best part is that is quick!! No 2 hour training videos here!! Ha-ha. Take a look and sign up, I would love to see you each morning!

## Free "Fierce Abs" Video Series

This book is accompanied by a Free 3-part video series entitled, *"Fierce Abs"*. The video series consists of 3 free videos which highlight various workout techniques in this book that I created to help you achieve your abs goals. Whether it's a ripped six pack, tightening and toning your mid-section, or just losing a few pounds this workout will help you get there.

It is totally free and I wanted to offer full length workouts so you could follow along. If you prefer not to workout at home you can always watch the videos and incorporate some of my ideas into your routine.

Each video in the series corresponds to Chapter 7 and Chapter 8.

To get instant access to this videos now click this link: http://bit.ly/10WpHog or type it into your address bar.

You'll need to enter your first name and your email address so I can send you the videos but once you do that I'll send you the first video right away. You will receive videos 2 and 3 within the next few days. You can't do 3 workouts in one day!! :)

Please know that your email is completely safe, I don't share anyone's info EVER! At the bottom of every email is a link to discontinue future emails as well.

At the end of the 3rd workout I'll give you the opportunity to work out with me for 2 whole weeks and get "deep dive" training via video, so make sure you look out for that.

So before you go any further, make sure you click here http://bit.ly/10WpHog to get instant access to my free 3 part video series and let's help you get your own *Fierce Abs*!

# Chapter 1: The Abdominal Muscles and their Functions

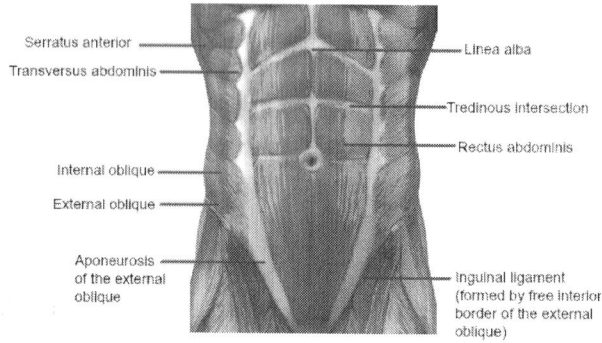

The abdominal muscles ("Abs" in this book) are a group of 6 muscles that attach to several places on your ribcage at the top and to various attachments on your pelvis at their lower extremities. They allow movement of and support the core (chest & back). They are one of the major groups of core muscles.

Abdominal muscles have several functions. They provide postural support and they also function to define your form. For example, the most external abdominal muscle, the rectus abdominus, gives the 6-pack-ab effect, desired by some, when it is exercised and built to a high degree of size and definition. The deeper and closer to the spine a particular abdominal muscle is, the greater its effect on body posture it will have. Having a strong, well-toned set of abs is a big factor that lends itself appreciably to a healthy back, good posture, good looks and good health in general.

The 6 Abdominal Muscles:

The deeper inside the body a particular abdominal muscle is located, the more powerful effect it will have, and therefore, it will have a greater capacity for stabilizing and maintaining a healthy, properly postured and formed spine. From the deepest to the shallowest (closest to the skin) the abdominal muscles are:

Transverse Abdominal - This muscle is the deepest of the 6 abdominal muscles. It wraps around your trunk from front to back and it contains and supports the organs located there. The fibers of this muscle run horizontally. Think of this muscle as a natural back support belt.

The transverse abdominal assists in breathing, helping the exhalation process by bringing the bottom of the ribcage closer to the spine, forcing air out of the lungs.
It also provides stability to the trunk and the organs located there as well as stability to the trunk during lateral flexion.

At the front the transverse abdominal muscle attaches to the linea alba which tends to lose its strength during pregnancy. Strengthening the transverse abdominal muscle after pregnancy is a good way to restore strength to the linea alba. (Note: When the linea alba is weak, lordosis is increased.

You can get a feeling for how this muscle works when you cough or laugh, paying attention to your abdominal area when you do.

Internal Obliques - These are a pair of deep abdominal muscles. They are situated just above the transverse abdominal muscle. The muscle fibers of the internal obliques connect from several points on or near the front of the hip bone and extend to the lower rib cage and the connective tissue of the rectus abdominus. The fibers from both the left and right muscle groups run in a direction such that they look like an inverted "V".

The lowest parts of the internal obliques work together with the transverse abdominal muscle to hold in and support the organs in the abdomen. The upper and lateral (side) parts of these muscles allow forward and lateral flexion and rotation of the spine, assist in supporting the contents of the abdomen and they also assist in breathing.

The internal obliques work with other abdominal muscles to perform some of these actions, especially lateral flexion and rotation of the spine.

External Obliques - These are two abdominal muscles that lie just above the internal obliques. Whereas the internal oblique muscle fibers run in an inverted "V" from the lower ribs to the front of front of the pelvic bones, the external obliques run in a "V". If you traced your forearms when your hands are in your pockets, this basically defines the lay of the external obliques.

These muscles are used in flexing the trunk forward, supporting the abdominal contents, breathing (especially exhalation), to rotate the ribcage and pelvis in opposite directions, tilt the pelvis and laterally flex the spine.

Some of these movements involve other abdominal muscles, especially for the rotational and lateral flexion motions.

Rectus Abdominis - This muscle is also commonly referred to as the Rectus Abdominus muscle. It is the most superficial of the six abdominal muscles (i.e. it lies "on top" of all the others). It runs from the front of the rib cage to the front of the pelvis, connecting to the pubis symphysis. Its main function is to flex the spine forward.

This is the "6 pack muscle"; although all abdominal muscles must be trained and developed properly to achieve a 6 pack tummy, this muscle is the most visible and, after getting rid of your abdominal fat, you can choose to just tone it as the front piece to your fit abdominal area or work it more to get any level of a "ripped" look.

## Chapter 2: The Abs You Already Have

In the just the first chapter of this book I am happy to present you with some very good news: You have abs! Everyone does; and as one of the core muscle groups, your abs are probably better developed than you may think, even if you may not be able to see them--yet. You have all six muscles shown in the illustration and described above. Since all these muscles are used in day-to-day activities they may already be pretty nicely built, just waiting for you to shed that fat and show them to the world.

In the coming chapters I will outline some exercises that you can follow, incorporate into your own workout, or use in conjunction with any of my workout programs including Fierce Abs to develop your own routines. The idea is to enjoy yourself and have fun with it. We will also review various foods to eat and foods to avoid and why. I will also begin to offer you replacement foods that you can begin to incorporate into your diet so you don't feel hungry and without foods that are acceptable.

The two most detrimental enemies to the abs you already possess are poor posture and belly fat. Further, toning your abs and reducing the abdominal fat that keeps them hidden will be two things that this book will also focus on. Proper posture, while standing or sitting can, by itself, vastly improve how your abs look to the world. Proper diet and exercise will melt away the layers that keep your natural abs hidden. The chapters on exercise cover sculpting and strengthening of your abdominals as well as exercises to strengthen your postural muscle groups, such that without conscious effort, they hold you in correct posture all the time. Exercise is divided into two general types: Strength-building and Cardiovascular.

## Chapter 3: A Look in the Mirror

If you have a full-length mirror, great. Go stand in front of it now, naked. Stand as you normally would, relaxed. Don't try to make yourself look better when you first see your body in the mirror. Pretend you are just going about normal day-to-day activities for the moment.

Look at yourself from the front and from both sides. What do you see? You may have varying degrees of excess body fat, a lot of it being in your abdominal area. You may notice, especially from the side that your posture, when relaxed, allows your spine to curve unnaturally. Assess your body. Note things such as how you hold your head. Is your neck in alignment with the rest of your back? Does your back curve like an "S"? Touch, press and pinch various areas of your body to get a general idea of the amount of body fat that lies over different muscle groups.

Now, imagine a cable connected to the top of your head. That cable is being pulled straight up and your body follows. Straighten your spine until you achieve just the normal slight curves that it's supposed to have when extended properly. Align your neck with your upright back so your head is looking straight forward. Pull your shoulders back and up. Pull in your abdominal muscles to a comfortable degree. Adjust your pelvis so that your abs and lower back muscles pull it into a balanced alignment. Look at yourself again. Guaranteed you look different from when you first stepped in front of the mirror. You look taller, slimmer, more fit. You look better.

Of course, maintaining this posture will not be possible once you forget about controlling all the muscles that make you look like this. Without conscious effort you will begin to slouch again, forget to hold your tummy in and if you come back to your mirror after ten minutes all the effects will have vanished. This is why you will need to train all those muscle groups you used to get that instantaneous "better look" so that even when you're not thinking about them, they are toned and strong enough to keep you in that posture naturally. After years of being in the fitness industry and paying attention to my body, I have been able to do this all day long. I naturally tighten my abdomen all day and night long without even thinking about it. Nevertheless, like anything else, it takes time, effort, and you must constantly repeat it.

Now, make notes about the features you want to change. You may already have low body fat but your posture is off or may have great posture but want to get rid of the flabby areas. Start a journal. This is Day One. Write down what you want changed – if you are a Fierce Abs member you can make notes using the fitness assessment sheet and the goal sheet.

## Chapter 4: Understanding Your Body

You know your body well. You've spent your whole life inside it. You may be able to exercise a little and show results right away or you may eat one slice of pizza a year and can never seem to be able to slim down. In this chapter we will discuss basic body types, metabolism and the effects of age on metabolism and its other effects on your body.

Your Body Type:

There are three, long accepted major body types: The ectomorph, the endomorph and the mesomorph. More detailed body types that are being used more recently are also described below. In general, however, as we age our metabolism slows down, leading to retention of more calories than we used to be able to burn even without exercising. Knowing your basic physiology and how it has changed over the years will give you a better idea of how to set your goals, which is the next chapter in this book.

Ectomorphs are naturally skinny, slim in limb, hip and torso. They have high metabolic rates and usually have a small skeletal structure (although they may be tall) and not much muscle mass. These are the types of folks who "can eat anything they want and not gain a single pound."

Endomorphs are naturally bulky and usually classified as overweight due to a low metabolic rate. Large bone structure is common and, depending on their height, can look more or less like mesomorphs, although they usually have a lot of excess fat, mostly in their torso, hips and thighs. Endomorphs have a hard time losing weight even if they eat a normal, healthy diet. They need extra exercise to burn off calories that their metabolism does not burn.

Mesomorphs are in between these two general body types. They usually have good muscle development and size even if they never hit the gym and don't generally have to watch what they eat to maintain a pretty good body--until they get older.

No matter what body type you have as you get older you will usually retain more weight and build more reserves of body fat as a result of your metabolism slowing down. Some ectomorphs end up with big bellies when they hit thirty-something.

We are ruled by our genetic code, which evolved to make sure that we stayed alive long enough to reproduce and raise our young until they themselves were old enough to do so. We are hard wired to crave foods that are high in sugar, fat and salt to ensure that we have enough energy and mineral reserves to get through lean periods. Although, with that said, our ancestors had a much more active life and burned off energy that a modern lifestyle stores as fat. Still, when humans reach their 30's our body somehow knows that we have fulfilled our evolutionary duty and begins to store more fat as we are no longer young enough to hunt as much and have to make more efficient use of whatever nutrients we take in. But just as our genes force us to crave calories, we can force ourselves to take measures to eat healthier and exercise more. It doesn't help either that there are all kinds of "added" injected hormones and steroids in our foods making us more over weight and more addicted to the bad food as well. And all the things that ensure that we have an effortless lifestyle is a big culprit too. We have everything we need to not move from the couch.

The three body types given above are basic generalizations. Everyone is unique in genetic makeup and if we add in the factor of your age, if you have just given birth, etc. we end up with a very wide spectrum of body types. As an example, some ectomorphs might be reading this because their genetic makeup, age, recent pregnancy or any combination of these has them there with their normal lithe body but with a bunch of unwanted flab covering up what used to be some pretty good abs; and that paunch doesn't seem to go away as easily as an extra pound or two used to almost like magic. This book has chapters that deal specifically with each body type, and some more specific ones are given below, as well as things like the slowed metabolism of the middle-aged and exercises that are targeted to new moms.

More Specific Body Types:

Type 1 - This is our typical ectomorph build with narrow hips and shoulders. You've probably been described by your friends as "lanky". Usually, the type 1 body will store most of its fat in the abdominal area--the worst place for it to be when you want your abs to shine through. If you do want to gain a little weight so as not to look like a stick figure, increase your cup size, etc. you generally will have a hard time doing this. Even if you do put on weight, as mentioned, it will not spread evenly but land in front of and to the sides of your abs. Further, type 1 bodies have a difficult time building muscle mass.

    A typical recommended workout for your body type would involve cardio to blast at any abdominal fat and muscle building exercises for your shoulders, arms, butt and chest along with your targeted ab exercises. Since your bone structure is narrow, you will need to build muscle to define wider shoulders and a more rounded rear. Toning your pectoral (chest) muscles will lift your breasts in case they do increase in size so they will not sag. This is especially true, but normal, for pregnant women and new mothers whose cup size increases due to hormones and breast milk content.

Your general exercise routine will be to use relatively heavy weights if you do use them; please see the chapter on adding weights to training. Using heavier weights at lower reps builds muscle mass (size). As a type 1 you will probably have muscles that are pretty well toned, but as mentioned, need to build mass for definition and a more curvy physique. The same is true for your targeted ab workout; you will probably need to add weight to define your abs as your body type will be reluctant to increase their size and definition.

Type 2 - You have pretty thin arms and legs with not much muscle mass but have excess fat around your abdominal area. You tend to gain weight easily, especially around your midsection; but you also build muscle mass pretty fast.

You'll need a good cardio routine to get rid of that abdominal fat--and keep it off. This and a proper diet will expose your abs that you will be building in the meantime with targeted exercise. If your shoulders and butt are narrow and small, exercise with weights is recommended to fill these areas out. If you're happy with your narrow frame you can just concentrate on toning your slim muscles and may want to concentrate mainly on your butt and abs to get good definition over those two areas.

Type 3 - You have a small upper body and a disproportionately larger lower half. You tend to have larger muscles in your hip, thigh and butt areas, built around a larger frame there, especially wider hips in proportion to your shoulders. You probably have difficulty building mass on your upper body but will usually build muscle quite easily on your lower half.

You will need cardio to eradicate all the fat on your lower body. Cardio that involves a lot of upper body movement is recommended as opposed to lower body cardio, such as jogging or cycling, so that you get your upper body muscles toned and built more. Further, you may want to consider adding weights to your upper body exercises, whether doing cardio or muscle building, to balance your naturally heavier set lower area. Since your lower body tones and builds muscle quite readily, upper body concentration should be your target; your lower body will get toned and built to a good size since most exercises involve many muscle groups, drawing from the lower body even if you are doing flys or presses and other similar exercises.

Type 4 - Your body type has wide hips and shoulders but a narrow waist. Generally, you have an easy time adding muscle to your arms, chest, legs, butt and hips but you also tend to store fat in those areas as well. Your waist may be slim but either because of muscle definition or a little extra layer of fat, your abs may not show through. You need to do cardio to lose fat all over and mainly target your abs when doing muscle-building exercises.

Metabolism:

Metabolism is easy to define but can be tricky to understand. Basically, it is the rate at which your body works (burns calories) and is almost always measured as a resting metabolic rate (i.e. while you are not performing any activity).

Typically, an endomorph (see above) has a low metabolic rate. This is just that person's normal metabolic rate and they burn fewer calories per unit of time than an ectomorph, who has a higher natural metabolic rate. To illustrate, let's say we counted how long it would take two people to burn all the calories from a spoonful of sugar. One is an ectomorph and the other an endomorph and they are both female and both weigh 180 pounds. Both eat the spoon of sugar--about 23 calories each--and just sit there until all the calories are burned. A mesomorph or the average person would burn all these calories in about 18 minutes (We will discuss these calculations later). The ectomorph, depending on how much faster her metabolic rate is will burn them in about 16 minutes, maybe less, just by sitting there, her body performing its basic life support. The endomorph may take up to 20 minutes or more to burn the 23 calories just sitting there. Since the average person eats an average meal with about the same amount of calories, we can now see why endomorphs have more problems with excess fat. Any sugar, amino acids (from protein) or phospholipids (from fat) not burned for energy get converted back to fat and stored where your body type dictates.

    With this information it seems easy to lose weight--just don't eat those spoons of sugar, right? Well, this is one of the tricky things about metabolism. When your body senses that it is not getting any calorie input your metabolism slows down. Your brain thinks that you haven't been able to find food. Recall the earlier section where I touched on the topic of our genetic code ruling us. When our body thinks that it is not going to be able to get its regular supply of calories it goes into low gear. Your metabolism slows down and even an ectomorph's metabolic rate will resemble that of an endomorph. This is the main reason that "crash diets" don't work. You keep reducing your calorie intake and your body responds, as it is coded to do, by slowing your metabolism more and more--and even trying to store more fat--in an effort to keep you alive until you catch another wooly mammoth. (I call it the cave man days; I have talked about this stuff in my blogs and on my Facebook Fan Page. The less you eat the more your body goes into caveman mode not knowing when it will eat again so it holds onto everything and stores as fat.)

This is why diets (a word I do not like) have to be planned properly. Your body has to be satisfied that it is not in danger of starving. Thus, you eat foods that both satisfy your Genetic Dictator and do not go straight from "lips to hips". Although even the best planned diet will have little effect without exercise. The combination of proper nutrition and exercise will be discussed in a later chapter, after you have assessed yourself and set your goals.

Metabolism also slows down for other reasons, a major one being your age. Generally, as we finish the growth spurt of puberty where we are burning lots of calories to grow larger, our metabolism slows down and we start putting on weight. This is especially true for women as they are now mature enough to reproduce and women will not come into estrus unless they have a certain percentage of body fat. Many female athletes with extremely low body fat percentages, even if they are sexually mature at ages such as 16 or 17, do not menstruate because they don't meet the minimum body fat requirement that your genes set to be able to get pregnant.

There are other reasons, many very technical and specific, even down to the individual, why metabolism slows down; however, here we have the two main reasons that almost all of us have to deal with day-to-day. As a bonus for signing up for my free daily video tips at www.FierceMinute.com I will email you a free calorie calculator that you can use to help determine proper calorie intake based on your gender and measurements.

**Chapter 5: Set Your Goals**

Most of you reading this book would like to lose weight in addition to improving your muscle tone, and, possibly, size. Some of you will have tried to do this before and will have had varying degrees of success. You might be frustrated and wondering if this is the book that will finally get you in shape. Well, it's not. Let me explain...No book, exercise program, diet or fitness coach is going to get you in shape; but do you know what will? You.

Diets can be cheated on or given up on. Exercise programs, gym memberships and that ab machine in your closet can be quit. It's not because they don't work; it's because you did not work them. However it's not enough to say that most people don't stick to their weight loss and exercise regimen--you have to know why.

To get to the root of the "why" you need to answer some other questions. The first one would be: Do you really want to lose weight and achieve fierce abs? Now, all of you will say yes to this, so a follow-up question is in order: What are you doing to achieve this? Do you do cardio at least 5 times a week? Do you do any type of strength training at least two days a week? Do you consistently work on your flexibility, both for its own sake as well as to do more types of exercise? Do you take the stairs whenever you can instead of an escalator or an elevator, walk whenever you can, move around as much as possible and keep active? When not on a set diet do you eat healthy meals and count calories? These and numerous other questions pertaining to a healthy lifestyle are at the core of the answer to that question, "Why?"

Hopefully, after answering these questions you begin to see the answer. "Getting in shape" is not about planning, learning the latest new "breakthrough" exercise or setting a menu and making a "healthy" shopping list--it's about Doing. While all the above are precursors to getting in shape, it is not what you want to do, not what you think you should do, not what you will do. It is what you are doing now.

Thus, it seems that the real question is not whether or not you really truly want to lose weight and get those fierce abs. The more poignant question is what are you doing, right now, to get them. It's a much more difficult question to answer but you know what? It's easier to do something about it so that the answer comes naturally. Here's how: Stop reading at the end of this paragraph. Get down on the ground right now, wherever you are and whatever you're wearing and do any ab exercise you know. Do it until you feel your abs burn. Any exercise that is safe for you is fine. If you can't do an ab exercise due to recent surgery or any other reason choose another exercise. No excuses. Work out until you feel the burn NOW; then come back.

There. You've done something. You are now a Doer. As you go through the rest of this book and as you set your goals and plan out your routine, never forget to "do". This brings me to one final point before we get into the details of goal-setting. What will you "Do" after you've achieved your fierce abs? Have you thought of this? Will you stop doing? You've achieved your goal, after all. Do you have to continue? Yes. Why? Because getting fit and staying fit are different goals. Your primary goal should be to stay fit, not just to get there and have to repeat the process all over again because you stopped doing.

Many experts call this making a "lifestyle change"-- I call it Life. Whether you lose weight because it is a risk to your health, to look better and feel better about your body, or any other reason, don't put blinders on until you reach your goal. Rather, enjoy the process. Make your new nutrition plan, new exercise routine--your new life--

make it enjoyable. It should never become a task, a chore to get through so you can get on with enjoying your life. It should be the enjoyment of your life itself. Think of it this way, as an allegory to your life as a whole. Have you ever thought like this: It is your last day alive and you are happy because you have reached your goal? You worked hard, did your best, and now that it is over you are content in the fact that you have succeeded. I don't think any of us view life this way, our goal having been reached on our last day on this Earth. Most of us naturally enjoy the journey; and this is what we have to focus on more concerning the exercise and diet facets of our lives. Don't focus on the destination, that last day you have, whether or not you've achieved a six-pack or not as you lay in bed. Enjoy the journey; take pleasure in the "getting there". Don't limit your triumph to the "one day when I finally get those Fierce Abs"; relish the entire life you lead creating those fierce things--and keeping them. I talk about this all the time and wrote a great article on this; have a look here http://bit.ly/WqWyKy. I think you will enjoy it!

    Your journey started when you got on the floor and exercised and felt the burn a little while back. Keep enjoying that journey. Enjoy your life!

    Now that you've become a person of action, we will now make your action plan. When I said your primary goal is to Do, I didn't mean that you should go off and diet, exercise and do random things to get in shape. We set our goals now and figure out the best possible way to achieve them, and to enjoy the entire process and everything that comes after. In fact, you've done quite a lot already. Your notes (remember I advised you to start a journal earlier) should look something like this:

Day One:

I can see how I can improve my posture just by standing straight and pulling my shoulders back. When I tighten my abs even just a little and stand tall it looks like I've already lost 5 pounds! Now, what I will do is exercise all the muscles I feel that I am working to maintain this good posture so that they will hold this great-looking me in this position automatically. I need to work my shoulders and upper back as well as my hip flexors to maintain a properly aligned spine. My core, especially my abs need toning and strengthening to keep this tummy tucked in while I get rid of this flab with cardio.

I have the basic endomorph body type with most of my extra fat around my lower torso and thighs. (Note to Self: Get a good all-around cardio routine going but focus on some weight training on the muscles mentioned above and for general upper body strength building. I will look more balanced if my narrow shoulders fill out and match my hips when they get to a good trim size.)

I turned 30 almost 6 months ago. My metabolism isn't as fast as it used to be and was never really supercharged. Along with focused cardio workouts I will walk to the grocery and take the stairs at work to the fifth floor where my office is. That will add to my daily burn level; also, I have already repositioned some things in the house to make me move around more while I cleared a workout area that usually has some stuff on it but I can easily move it out of the way to exercise and put it back after--extra calories burned!

Hello again! I left for a bit and just did some bending exercises. I can't touch my toes yet--but I will--and I did feel my abs working and burning to pull me to bend low; the front of my thighs also got a good stretch...Back to my plan.

I checked out the chapter where it showed me what my weight target should be. I'm 160 now and with my height I need to lose 25-30 pounds. I also looked at the section on HIIT and I like it! I can burn a lot in less time. Work is pretty hectic now so I'm glad I found out about this. I also have a long commute but I now know exercises that I can do while driving or sitting on the bus--or at my desk even :) Ok, we're getting this together.

*Yes, I am planning now; but I have just become a Doer. As I sit here getting this plan organized I am making sure to sit straight and am exercising my abs by holding them in for a ten count. I just did three reps in the last two paragraphs! Burn, Baby, Burn!!!*

*(Note to Self: Download that song I just heard on the radio. That'll put some pump into my chest flys...Ok, now to the kitchen to do a food inventory and then back here to put together a fierce upper body workout routine. gotta do it quick, still have to cook dinner. I was gonna get takeout but I have enough time to get this outline done and make a fierce meal ;) ...'til tomorrow and it's already marked:*

*Day Two:*

Specific Weight Loss Goals:

    Each of us has different reasons for losing weight and some of us will need or want to lose more than others. We may have been told by our doctor to lose 5-10% of our weight for health reasons, would like to lose 30 pounds to fit into our leather breeches from the 90's-- a whole spectrum. Basically, the main consideration when setting a target weight and the time you will give yourself to get there is that it has to be realistic. This will keep you motivated because you know that it is an achievable goal and you will be able to see results every few days by stepping on the scale. However, using the scale is too often is also something I do not recommend as a way to telling you if you are making progress. Why? Because your body is always naturally fluctuating so it's impossible to get a real read unless you take progress photos and stand in the mirror to check your achievements. You may want to, or have to, lose a hundred pounds, but setting a goal to do that in 60 days is tantamount to setting your goal to "fail". Check out my Fierce Minute tips to help you better understand this, http://bit.ly/WVdhGC and my other tip http://bit.ly/WYIzLe. The first thing you need to do is look at some commonly used parameters for weight loss. Knowing this information will guide you in setting a realistic goal. Some of the calculations given below are based on the average person. You may have a faster or slower metabolism or other factors that will change these figures. One you have your basic calculations and measurements it would be a good idea to consult your family doctor and discuss your plan. Your doctor will be able to advise you on fine tuning the numbers, with goal-setting in general and, most importantly, remind you of any health considerations you need to keep in mind when setting up your nutrition plan and your exercise routine. Conducting a simple online search will give you pages with free calculators for the computation of the needed information below or you can go to www.FierceMinute.com and as a bonus for signing up for my free daily video tips and I will email you a free calorie calculator that you can use to help determine proper calorie intake based on your gender and measurements.

    First, figure out your Basal Metabolic Rate (BMR). This is the amount of calories your body burns just to stay alive and a good one will take into consideration your typical activity level for an average day such as "seated at a desk", "moderate housework", "heavy lifting", etc. If you consume this amount of calories every day you will maintain your present weight. Cutting it by 500 calories a day will lower your weight by 1 pound a week, and it is not recommended to lower it by more than 750 calories a day because your metabolism will probably slow down, as discussed in the previous chapter. For every 500 calories a day that you consume above this amount, you will gain an additional pound a week.

Next, calculate your Body Mass Index (BMI) – a simple Google search will yield numerous free calculators. Anything 25 and over is considered overweight so you'll need to plan to drop down into the healthy range (18.5 to 24.9). You might only need to lose 5 pounds to hit 24.9 but if, for example, you really want to start wearing those really tight jeans again you might want to drop down to the lower range of healthy BMI, somewhere around 19-21; However, going down to a BMI below 18.5 is considered being underweight and may have health risks of its own.

Now, measure your waist, after exhaling, at the narrowest point between the bottom of your ribs and the top of your pelvis; then, with your heels together, measure around the largest part of your hips and buttocks. Divide your waist measurement by your hip measurement. A healthy waist-to-hip ratio for women is .86 and below and, for men, it is .95 or less.

Finally, take into consideration your abdominal girth which is a waist measurement taken at belly button level. Measurements of more than 35 inches for women and 40 for men are too high.

Take all this information into consideration but remember that these are based on values obtained from the average person. For example, you may have a Type 4 body, meaning your waist size may not be a good indicator. Focus more on your BMI rather than the waist-to-hip ratio and abdominal girth. If you have a lot of muscle mass, this can throw off your BMI measurement, muscle being heavier than fat. Your calculated BMI might be over 24.9 but you actually have a normal body fat percentage and are thus not overweight but actually well-muscled. Your waist-to-hip ratio will usually show you if your BMI is off.

Present this information to your doctor when making your plan and setting your goals and the two of you can fine tune your goals to make a personalized plan. Here is a sample information sheet that you could present to your doctor:

December 21

Age: 29
Basic body type: Typical Ectomorph when growing up, now, Type 2
Height: 5'4"
Weight: 160 lbs.
BMR: **1,436 calories/day**
BMI: 27.5
Waist and Hips: 34/32
Waist-to-hip Ratio: 1.06
Abdominal Girth: 38.5

Notes: I tallied up my average daily calorie intake and it's over 1800! That means I'm gaining almost a pound a week =( I have a thyroid condition and Dr. Darrin said my meds may slow down my metabolism; I'm also pushing 30. My limbs are still pretty thin but I'd like to lose this gut I've had for a couple of years. I would like to hit and maintain a weight of 120 (which would put my BMI at 20.6)--lower end of the healthy range...but I have this killer dress I want to get into again! It fit real nice when I was 120-125 :) So, I gotta drop 40 pounds. If I cut 400 calories a day through a better diet and another 700 thru exercise, I will do this in 29 weeks, losing about 1.4 pounds a week--just in time for my 30th birthday--where I will wear that dress!! Since my BMR is just over 1400 calories I should cut most of the 1100 through exercise, mostly cardio to kill the tummy with focus on my chest muscles to give my breasts a lift ;) This is almost a 7 month plan so if I can stick to it that long I should probably be able to continue.

Proposed diet modifications - Replace my usual two sodas a day with fruit juice (-160 kcal); one egg with breakfast and supplement with fruit (-80 kcal); have my one glass of wine every other night rather than nightly (-45 kcal); I can eat more baked and boiled meals and if I really want something fried I can cut the fat from oil with non-stick coating. This will get me down by my target 400 kcal for diet.

> Exercise plan - I'm lucky. I can walk to work almost every day of the year. It's a pretty long walk but it will burn about 350 calories even if I take it easy. I will do extra cardio and strength training for half an hour every other day; that's another 675 kcal taken care of. 75 more to go...I'll eventually be able to walk faster and could take a bit off with my diet. In the meantime I'll do extra jumping jacks and jump rope on Sundays; ten minutes each will do it, and give me an energy boost so I can enjoy my Sundays!

This is looking like a great plan! This lady has a BMR of only 1,436 kcal and her goal is to lose 40 pounds in just over 6 months. She has to cut down/burn 1,100 calories a day to do that (That's almost half the BMR of a 6-foot tall male!). But, as you can see, by giving herself enough time, making easy diet modifications and working exercise into her daily schedule, she will meet her goal.

After reading through this book you will be able to fine-tune your goals as well as make a personalized diet plan and workout routine. Feel free to skip forward and back to chapters and sections if you want more information on what you are doing now or if you want to check something you've read for confirmation. The following chapter gives recommended workouts based on your general body type. Modify any variable you want and add any other exercises given in later chapters to sculpt the body that you want--and that you have already begun to create.

Would you like to be showcased on one or all of my websites? If you are starting your journey and want to make your progress known to the world you can go to my testimonials page at http://bit.ly/WL382s and submit and before and after photos. I would love to see you progress from beginning to end!!

## Chapter 6: Building on Your Foundation

Here are some basic workouts by body type. Please refer to the chapters and sections on weights and cardio training for more specific information. Illustrations are provided to assist you with proper form during the exercise.

Sample Workout for Type 1 Bodies:

These exercises will add form to and tone your butt, chest, arms and shoulders. For women, toning your chest muscles will lift your breasts higher. Do three sets of six to eight reps for each exercise. Since you have a naturally lean body type, do 30-45 minutes of the cardio of your choice a minimum of three times a week. Your focus should be maintenance over burning a lot of calories unless, due to factors discussed in previous sections you have fat covering your abs.

Weighted Squats - Works your legs and butt. Stand with feet shoulder-width apart and hold your weights near your shoulders. Squat down until your thighs are parallel to the floor. Your center of gravity should be pressing down through your heels. Bring your elbows to your knees at the bottom of the squat then press back up through your heels using your front thigh muscles.

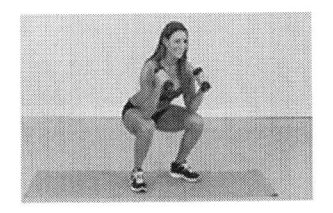

Bench Press - Works your chest, shoulders and arms. Lie face-up on a ball or bench; a large sofa cushion will also work. Hold your weights with arms straight and hands facing up. Bring your weights down by bending your elbows out to your sides until your hands are at chest level. Press up and repeat. If you want an advanced version, check out my video tip here: http://bit.ly/10JlVcj.

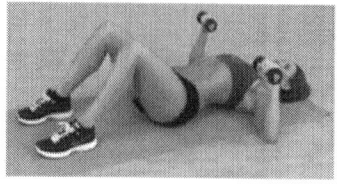

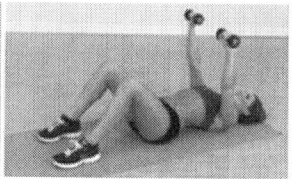

Sample Weekly Workout Plan:

Monday: Do strength-training
Tuesday: Day Off
Wednesday: Walk or jog vigorously outside or inside on a treadmill if you have one or the weather is not good; try for 3.5 to 6.0 mph and 5%+ incline for 30 mins; then do strength-training.
Thursday: Do your cardio workout of choice for 45 to 60 mins.
Friday: Do Strength-training.
Saturday: Day Off
Sunday: Walk for 30 to 45 mins at a quick rate (about 4.0 to 4.2 mph) for a maximum of 1 hour.
Sample Workout for Type 2 Bodies:

These compound exercises will tone your abs and sculpt your arms and legs. Since you also put on muscle quite quickly, use moderate to light weights, doing 3 sets of 12 - 15 reps for each exercise. To really blast fat, especially around your tummy, do cardio of your choice at least 3 days a week, 5 being most advantageous, working at a temperate to spirited pace for 30 to 45 minutes.

Squat Thrust with Push-Up - Works your legs, abs, chest, arms, butt, and shoulders. Stand with your feet shoulder-width apart. Put hands on the floor, and then kick your legs back into a proper push-up position. Do 1 push-up (on your knees if necessary), then hop feet forward between your hands. Repeat.

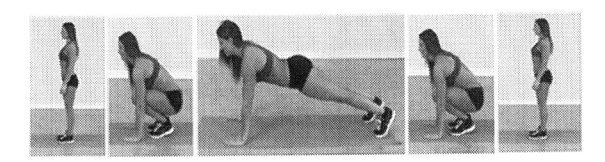

Standing Rotation Exercise - Works your Abs, back, shoulders, butt and legs. A medicine ball is best for this exercise but any sort of weights will do. Stand with feet shoulder-width apart and hold your weight close to your body at just below chest level. Engage your abdominal and other core muscles and maintain good posture, pulling your shoulder blades back without arching your lower back. Bring your weight up in front of you, elbows bent slightly, and rotate your torso in one direction. Don't lean into the rotation, maintain a straight spine and move your head in the same direction as the rotation. Hold the position for a few seconds and then return to center then rotate in the opposite direction. For a more intense workout, extend your arms fully, holding your weight far out from your chest at shoulder height.

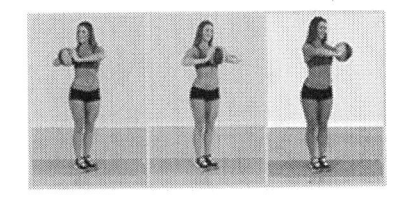

Tip for Rotation Exercises: Most people use their arms to move the weight from side to side. While this does exercise your arms and shoulders it does not target the muscles you want worked the most, your abs. The trick is to immobilize your arms at the shoulder and concentrate on twisting using your abs and your core. Pretend that your body, from the top of your head to your ribcage is paralyzed. Rotate by engaging your abs to do all the work.

Sample Weekly Workout Plan:

Monday: Walk rapidly (about 4.2 mph) for 45 mins to 1 hour; do strength-training.
Tuesday: Do interval training: After warming up, swap between 0% and 10% incline on a treadmill, 2 mins for each incline position, or find a moderately inclined hill if you want to work outside. Do this 5 times then cool down.
Wednesday: Do your favorite cardio for 30 to 45 mins.
Thursday: Walk quickly (3.8 to 4.0 mph) at a 5%+ incline for 45 mins; do strength-training.
Friday: Do your favorite cardio for 30 to 45 mins.
Saturday: Do strength-training.
Sunday: Day Off

Sample Workout for Type 3 Bodies:

Use heavier weights and fewer reps (around 6 to 8 per set) for your upper body exercises to build lean muscle mass and achieve proportionality with your lower body. For your lower body, use lighter weights and more reps (around 12 to 15 per set) to tone and sculpt healthy muscle mass on your lower body trouble areas. 3 sets of each exercise is recommended. Additionally, do cardio 5 times a week to burn lower body fat. Your best choices are workouts that burn calories while building upper-body endurance like kickboxing and rowing.

Lateral Raise - This works your shoulders. Stand with feet shoulder-width apart, holding your weights with your hands facing inwards, arms straight down. Raise your arms out to your sides up to shoulder height, keeping your elbows slightly bent and pinkie fingers higher than thumbs at the top of the raise. Hold for a couple of seconds then lower and repeat.

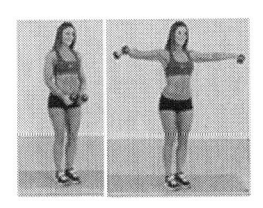

Squat/Lunge Combination - Works legs back and butt. Stand with your feet shoulder-width apart and your arms down at your sides. Step out to your left side with your left foot and squat down; keeping your weight over heels so not to lose your balance (you should feel your weight press down on the bottoms of your heels). Bring your right foot in next to your left foot. Now lunge behind you with your left foot, bending forward at the waist and touch your right ankle or instep of your foot with both hands. Return to start and repeat on the opposite side which completes one rep.

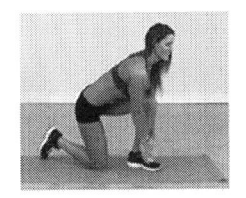

Sample Weekly Workout Plan:

Monday: Walk outdoors or on treadmill at the gym at a 5%+ incline at 4.0 mph for 45+ min.
Tuesday: Do your favorite cardio for 45 mins and do strength-training.
Wednesday: Day Off
Thursday: Do your favorite cardio for 45 to 60 mins and do strength-train.
Friday: Run and walk in intervals (HIIT). Try doing 6 sets and then cool down.
Saturday: Do your favorite cardio for 45 mins.
Sunday: Do strength-training.
Sample Workout for Type 4 Bodies:

Because you tend to gain muscle without difficulty, you'll notice increases in strength and endurance relatively quickly even if you're using medium weights. Do 3 sets of 10 reps for each exercise. To burn fat, try doing circuit training that combines your strength workouts with cardio bursts such as jumping jacks, jumping rope, high knees, or jogging/sprinting in place.

Front Raise with Triceps Press - Works your arms and shoulders. Stand with feet shoulder-width apart and hold your weights with hands facing down. Raise your arms to shoulder height; hold for a count of 1, then resume lifting your arms higher and over your head. Rotate your arms so your palms face inward and bend your elbows, lowering the weights behind your head. Straighten your arms to return to the start position and repeat.

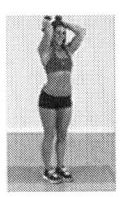

Reverse Lunge with Rotation - Works your obliques, butt and legs. Stand with your feet shoulder-width apart and hold your weights near your shoulders, hands facing each other. Lunge backwards with your left leg. Return to the starting position and lift your left knee as you rotate your torso to the left. Lower your leg, face forward and repeat for your right side. Also for a quick video tip check out http://bit.ly/WYIKGqt to really get you fired up!

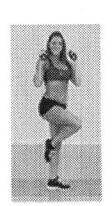

Your Workout Plan

Monday: Circuit training. Do the recommended strength workout, and add 2-minute cardio training such as HIIT (jumping jacks, etc.) between each strength exercise.
Tuesday: Walk outside or on the treadmill at 4 mph for 45+ mins or run at 6 mph for 30+ mins.
Wednesday: Day Off
Thursday: Do your favorite cardio for 30 to 45 mins and do strength training.
Friday: Day Off
Saturday: Circuit training like on Monday
Sunday: Do your favorite cardio for 45 - 60 mins and include a few 30-second sprints as cardio such as my HIIT exercises.

Additional Exercises for All Body Types:

Incorporate these six moves into your regular workouts to change things up a bit and avoid plateaus.
1. Floating Lunge - Works your legs, butt and abs. Hold your weights at your sides. Lunge forward with your right leg and bend your knee. Push your right foot to the left, toward your center line, balancing for just a second. Step back with your right foot coming into a reverse lunge and bring that foot left again to maintain balance along your center line. Repeat with your left leg to complete one rep.

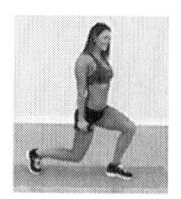

2. V-Sit with Chest Flys - Works your chest and abs. Sit with good posture on the floor with your knees bent and your feet flat on the floor while holding your weights close to your chest. Lean back slightly at the hips, keeping your abs engaged (tight and contracted), extending your arms to your front with your hands facing inward. Slowly swing your arms out to your sides at shoulder level while lowering your torso to about 45 degrees off the floor. Bring your arms and weights back in front of you, arms still extended. Bring your torso back up almost fully and repeat. I added this extra advanced version for the chest press and want to show you this on the stability ball for advanced versions. Watch here for advanced: http://bit.ly/XB9Fbr.

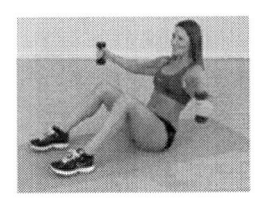

3. T-Stand Row - Works your upper back and abs. Stand with your feet shoulder-width apart, holding your weights at your sides. Lift your right leg behind you and lean forward from the hips until your body is parallel to the floor. Keep your arms extended downwards with your hands facing each other. Bring your arms up, elbows tucked near your ribs with arms close to your sides. Hold for a count then straighten arms back down slowly. Repeat, lifting your left leg; this is one rep.

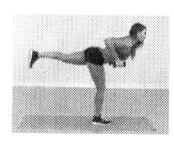

4. Side Lunge and Press - Works your shoulders and legs. Stand with your feet shoulder-width apart and point your toes outward. Hold your weights near your shoulders, with your elbows bent and hands facing each other. Lunge to your left with your left leg and press your right arm and weight straight above your head. Return to your start position as you lower your arm and then lunge with your right leg, pressing up with your left arm. This is one rep.

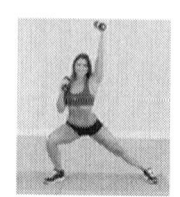

5. Bicep Curl/Front-Raise Combination - Works your shoulders and biceps. Stand with your feet shoulder-width apart and extend your arms to your sides while holding your weights in your hands. Slowly curl the weights toward your body and then bring your arms down out of the curl. Next, rotate your forearms so your hands face downwards; lift arms up, keeping elbows slightly bent outwards. Lower your weights and repeat the bicep curl portion and the front raise combination.

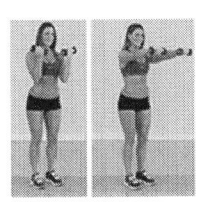

6. Balancing Triceps Kickback - Works your legs, butt and triceps. Stand with your feet shoulder-width apart, holding your weights at your sides and your hands facing in. Lift your right leg behind you and squat down halfway with your left leg, bending forward at the hips as you extend your arms back behind you, keeping your elbows near your sides. Bend your elbows and curl the weights toward your shoulders. Repeat, lifting your left leg back and half-squatting with your right leg. This is one rep.

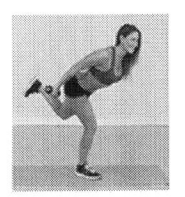

Nine Ab-targeting Exercises:

Tips for Ab Exercises: Abs are used every day and thus can be exercised every day, although every other day is usually enough. If you hit them hard you should be feeling the burn (and the pain) after 20 minutes. If you have to do 100 reps of any exercise before you feel the burn, you're really not getting much out of the exercise. You need to crank it up by performing the moves faster and/or with weights (or, with exercises like crunches and sit-ups, do them declined). You should be wincing in pain after 10-20 minutes and with a fierce workout like this done every other day, your abs will be toned, strong and ready to shine by the time you've melted away their outer shell of fat with your cardio routine.

1. Bird Dog Gets Down (Targets rectus abdominis, obliques, your back, and transversus abdominis)

    Get down on all fours. Raise your hips up and back as you straighten your elbows and knees to end up in an inverted V position. Lift one leg up and extended behind you. Keeping one leg lifted, move forward and bend your elbows again, lowering your hips to come to the pushup position, shoulders directly over your wrists. Hold for a couple of seconds and return to the inverted V position. Do 10-15 reps and then repeat the set with your other leg raised. Do 2-3 sets for each side.

    With your right leg raised, move your body forward to get into a full push-up position, your shoulders should be directly over your wrists. Hold for one count then return to the start position. Do 10 - 15 reps; repeat after switching sides and do 2 - 3 sets.

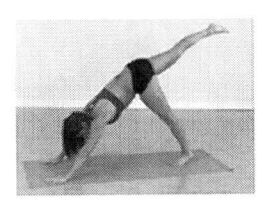

2. Tolasana with Blocks or Weights (Targets your obliques, transversus abdominis and rectus abdominis)

Sit on the floor with your knees bent and ankles crossed; place your hands flat on top of a yoga block or weights (or even piles of sturdy books) on either side of your body.
Straighten your arms and exhale as you tighten your abs to lift yourself including your butt and legs off the floor. Hold for 10 - 15 seconds, keeping your core tight. Lower slowly.
Challenge yourself: From your lifted position, try to extend your legs forward in midair as you hold the position. Try doing 6 reps, alternating the way you cross your legs.

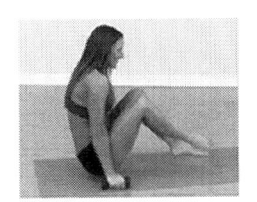

3. Side Plank (Targets your obliques, rectus abdominis, and transversus abdominis)

   Start in a regular push-up position with feet close together and balanced on the balls of your feet. Get your yoga block or a heavy book with your right hand and twist your body into the side plank: Shoulders and hips should be in line as mine are in my video, balancing on your palm and the outer side of your same-side foot (left hand, left foot). Raise your right arm, lifting the weight. Bring your right arm underneath your rib cage. Raise your arm again. Do 10 to 15 reps. Switch sides and repeat. Try doing 2 to 3 sets. For another fun advanced exercise click here http://bit.ly/VbZvyb.

4. Magic Carpet (Targets your obliques, rectus abdominis, and transversus abdominis)

   Get onto the floor in the regular push-up position. (Note: The floor should be uncarpeted and slippery) Balance on your hands and toes, arms extended and core engaged with a folded towel under your feet (for them to slide on). Squeeze your abs and bring your knees in toward your chest. To see how to do this with gliders click here http://bit.ly/14i0rqu, it's so tough but works so much of your body!

Challenge yourself: Keep your legs straight and lift your hips high into a pike position then bring feet toward hands, keeping hips high and arms and legs extended. Hold for a count of one and then return to start position. Try 3 sets of 10 reps and rest about 45 seconds between each set.

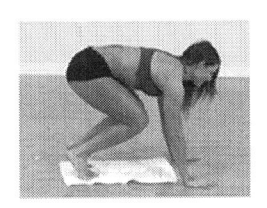

5. Pass the Block (Targets your transversus abdominis and rectus abdominis)

Lie face-up on the floor with your arms extended behind your head and both hands holding a yoga block or heavy book. Curl up by contracting your abs to reach your hands toward your toes, bending knees to place the weight between your feet. Holding the block (or whatever you are using) with your feet, lower your torso back down as you extend arms behind head and straighten out your legs. Reverse the motion, transferring the weight to your hands to complete 1 rep. and try doing 3 sets of 10 reps.

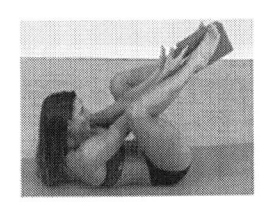

6. Wide-Legged Criss-Cross (Targets your obliques, rectus abdominis, inner thighs, transversus abdominis)

   Lie face-up on the floor with your hands behind your head, elbows bent out to your sides, and legs extended straight up, squeezing a yoga block or a book between your thighs. Curl your shoulders off floor by contracting your abs and rotate your torso to bring your left elbow toward your right side. Return to center and repeat, rotating in the opposite direction. Try doing 2 to 3 sets of 20 reps. Alternate sides.

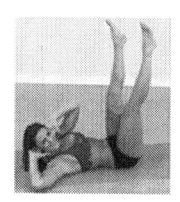

7. Balancing Act (Targets your transversus abdominis and rectus abdominis)

    Lie face up on the floor and bend your knees up to your chest to place a single yoga block or book on the soles of your feet (flex them so your soles face up); place your arms on the floor slightly out to your sides and slowly extend legs straight up, balancing the weight on your soles. Without rocking, use your abs to slowly lift your hips a few inches off mat and lower them again. Try doing 2 - 3 sets of 10 reps.

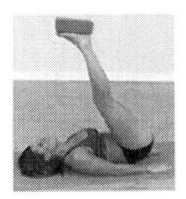

8. Lean Back (Targets your obliques, inner thighs, transversus abdominis, and rectus abdominis)

    Sit on the floor with knees bent, feet flat on the floor with one yoga block or book between your knees. Place your hands behind your head, elbows out, and extend your right leg forward and up. Lean back a few inches hold for a few counts then squeeze your abs to pull your torso back up.

Optional: Place a support behind your hips. Try doing 2 - 3 sets of 25 reps. Switch legs for each set.

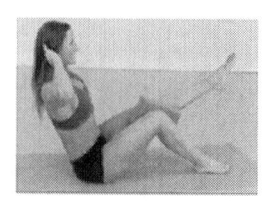

9. Warrior Curl (Targets your rectus abdominis, transversus abdominis, butt and obliques)

Place a yoga block or stacks of books shoulder-width apart on floor. Bend forward 90 degrees at your hips and place your hands on top of the blocks, shoulders aligned over wrists. Extend your left leg behind you until it is parallel to the floor with your toes pointing down. Squeeze your abs and arch your back as you bring your left knee toward your head. Try doing 10 reps. Switch legs and repeat doing 2 - 3 sets.

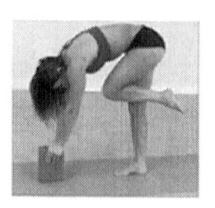

You should now have your goals and basic workout plan written down. Do the exercise set recommended for your body type, including the targeted abdominal exercises, but don't be afraid to change it up with the six other recommended exercises to avoid hitting a loss of weight. (Plateaus are discussed in more detail in a later chapter.) Remember, the general rule of thumb is that strength training will tone muscles, increase their size or both, variant on the amount of weight used and the number of reps done per set. Lighter weights and more reps are for endurance and toning and heavy weights with fewer reps build more mass. While exercises with weights will burn calories, it is cardio training that burns off excess fat in trouble areas. As you go through your routine, keep taking notes to help you determine the correct balance of strength training and cardio workouts for you. Keep fine tuning your regimen.

## Chapter 7: Extra Fierce Exercises

Here are ten fierce workouts that work your core and your abs really well. Incorporate them into your regular workout schedule as targeted ab exercises.

1. Side Plank Pulse:

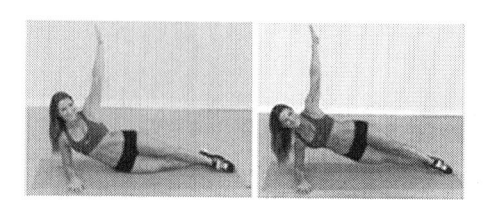

    Step 1 - Lie on a the floor on one side, stack your feet on top of each other and position your elbow directly under your shoulder. Exhale slowly, lifting your hips and torso off the ground keeping your abs and glutes contracted. Keep your left arm raised reaching towards the ceiling.

    Step 2 - Begin to lower and raise your hips towards and away from the ground in small movements. To make this exercise more difficult raise your upper leg a few inches off your bottom leg. This exercise works your deep core and stability muscles. Repeat exercise for 30-60 seconds then switch sides and repeat.

2. Jack Knife Pass Off (with Stabilty Ball):

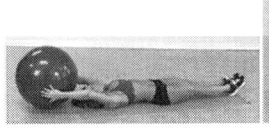

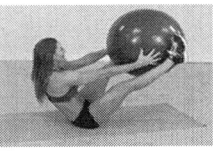

Step 1 - Lie on the floor with your legs spread out as wide as your stability ball and hold the ball behind your head with your arms stretched back.

Step2 - Squeeze your abs to lift your torso and legs into a "V" position (jack knife) and pass the ball to grip between your ankles, keeping your arms straight and swinging the ball towards your feet as you do this.

Step 3 - Slowly relax your abs and lay back down with the ball gripped between your feet and your arms extended behind your head. Repeat the jack knife motion and pass the ball to your hands again.

Fierce Video Tip for Lower Leg Raise - http://bit.ly/10SDA60

3. Reverse Stability Ball V-UP (can be done with or without a stability ball)

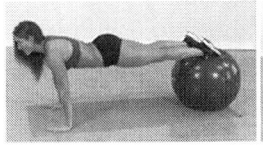

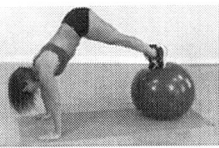

Step 1 - Place the stability ball behind you (or just get into the standard push up position if you're not using a ball). Place your lower legs on top of the ball and squeeze your core and glutes to maintain a straight posture parallel to the floor with your hands directly under your shoulders.

Step 2 - Squeeze your abs to lift your hips high up into the air in a reverse "V"; the tips of your toes should balance on top of the ball (or on the floor) and your hips should come up and forward almost directly above your head. Slowly lower back down, keeping your core engaged for posture and repeat.

4. Stability Ball Knee Tuck (Can be done without stability ball)

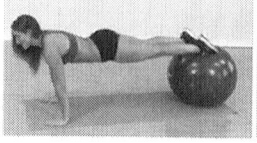

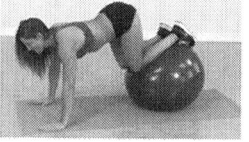

Step 1 - Get into a push up position with your lower legs on a stability ball if you're using one. Squeeze your abs and bend your knees to roll the ball and your thighs forward; your hips should move up slightly and your head should now be about a foot lower than your hips.

Step 2 - Keeping your arms straight under your shoulders the whole time, reverse the motion, straighten your back and keep your core engaged for good posture. Repeat.

5. Fierce Burpees:

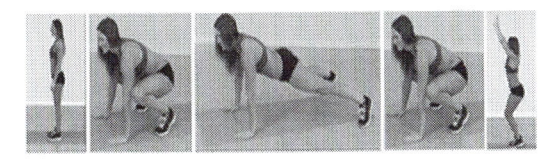

Description: I love burpees but I change the intensity up by changing the movements. Here is a great advanced burpee to try. The method described below is the "four count burpee" as it has four distinct steps.

Refer to the illustrations above as you follow the descriptive steps below:

Step 1 - Begin by standing with space in front of you for headroom and space behind you to extend your legs.

Step 2 - Drop to a squat position with your torso bent forward more and your arms extended downwards, hands flat on the floor. Keep feet as wide as hands (count 1).

Step 3 - - Kick both of your feet back and keep feet as wide as hands throughout in one quick motion, landing on your toes in a wide stance as if getting ready for a pushup (count 2).
Then bring your body all the way to the floor and push up for a full body pushup.

Step 4 - Bring your legs forward wide stance and quickly to return to the squat position (count 3).

Step 5 - Jump straight up as high as you can, extending your arms above your head (count to 4).

6. Advanced Mountain Climbers:

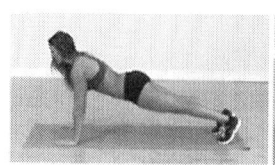

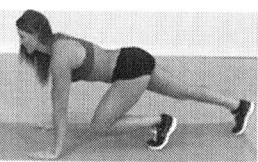

In this exercise you will get into a pushup position but bring one foot to the outside of your hand. Then as you bring it back to the center you then quickly switch your other foot to the other hand. That's one rep. You will go as fast as you can and stay wide.

7. Plank Press-Up:

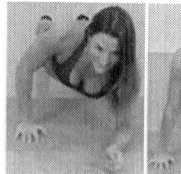

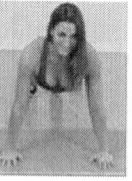

Get into the standard plank position. Move one arm at a time back (bending your elbows) to get ready for a push up. Do a push up and then return to the plank one arm at a time.

8. Single Arm/Leg Raise

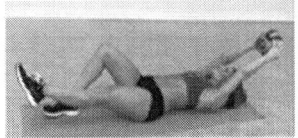

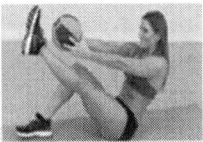

Lie down, face-up, with one knee bent and the other leg straight out. Hold a medicine ball behind your head, arms outstretched. Squeeze your abs and bring your torso and straight leg up in a "V" and swing your arms up over your head and forward to touch the ball to your foot. Repeat with the other leg bent.

9. Kettle Bell Swing (can be done with a dumbbell)

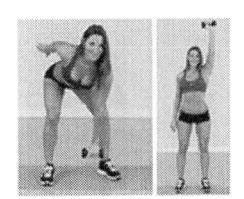

Feet shoulder width apart, bend at the knees slightly and hold your weight between your legs, torso bent forward and back straight. Straighten your knees and stand up straight while swinging the weight up in front of you and over your head, straightening your arm. Lower and repeat. Work both arms.

10. Advanced Knee Tuck

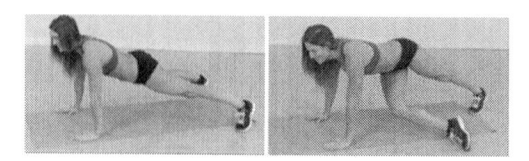

Start in a push up position with hips slightly elevated. Bring one knee forward near your chest and lower your hips. Turn your toes out to the opposite side of the leg you brought forward. Extend the leg back and repeat with the other leg.

## Chapter 8: The Big HIIT[1]

Not all cardio workouts are created equal. Have you ever heard of High Intensity Interval Training (HIIT)? In 1996, Izumi Tabata published his findings, the Tabata Protocol, after studying varying lengths of anaerobic workouts followed by short rest periods. Now known generally as HIIT, varying intense workout periods alternating with rest periods are employed by different trainers. HIIT is gaining popularity fast as an effective calorie burning cardiovascular routine that can be done in a fraction of the time of regular cardio workouts.

A typical HIIT workout involves a warm up period of low-intensity exercise, followed by six to ten bouts of high intensity exercise. In between the high intensity repetitions, medium intensity exercise is performed and the workout ends with a phase of cool down exercise. During the high intensity phases you should push yourself to near maximum intensity (e.g. sprint as fast as you can for the number of seconds for the phase). The medium exertion phases should be at about 50% of your maximum capable intensity. The number of repetitions and the length of each depends on the type of exercise chosen. One recommended target is to do at least six cycles of high and medium, 12 phases in all, and the entire HIIT workout should last at least fifteen minutes (but not more than twenty minutes and thirty minutes absolute maximum even if you're super fit).

The original protocol set a 2:1 ratio of time spent on maximum work to recovery periods (medium, or 50% exertion); for example, 30–40 seconds of hard sprinting phases with 15–20 second phases of jogging or brisk walking in between.

---

[1]HIIT Reference: http://bit.ly/14Y7J32

The original Tabata Protocol (IE1 Protocol) called for 20 seconds of high intensity exercise and 10 seconds of rest, done continuously for 4 minutes (8 cycles).

HIIT is an excellent way to maximize a cardio workout for people with limited time.

In 2009, the Little method was developed. This uses 3 minutes of warm-up then 60 seconds of intense exercise followed by 75 seconds of rest, repeated for 8–12 cycles.

HIIT is typically done by most people on a stationary exercise bike but no equipment is necessary. One can sprint in place or on a road or track. Some exercises incorporate stress release such as using a sledgehammer to pound on tires for the intense intervals.

Aerobic benefits:

Studies by Tabata, Tremblay and others have investigated the efficiency of this system compared to conventional endurance training routines. A study by Gibala et al. demonstrated that sprint interval training for two and a half hours produced similar biochemical changes in the subjects' muscles as did ten and a half hours of traditional endurance training. Similar benefits for endurance performance were also noted. According to a study by King, HIIT increases the resting metabolic rate (RMR) for an entire day (24 hours) following training due to excess post-exercise oxygen consumption, and may improve maximal oxygen consumption ($VO_2$ max) more successfully than doing just conventional long aerobic workouts. Tabata's 1997 study concluded that "intermittent exercise defined by the IE1 protocol may tax both the anaerobic and aerobic energy releasing systems almost maximally."

Athletic performance was also shown to benefit from high-intensity interval training with improvements recorded. For athletes that are already well-trained, performance improvements become hard to achieve and increases in the amount of training can potentially yield no improvement if traditional training methods are employed. Previous research shows that improvements in endurance performance can be achieved through HIIT for athletes who are already well-trained. A recent study by Driller showed an 8.2 second improvement in 2000 meter (2200 yards) rowing time following four weeks of HIIT in well-trained rowers. (This is a significant 2% improvement after a mere seven HIIT sessions.) The interval training used by Driller and his research group involved 8 x 2.5 minute work phases at 90% of $vVO_2max$, with recovery periods of differing lengths for each individual between each high intensity interval.

Metabolic benefits:

Long aerobic workouts have long been touted as the best way to lose fat. This is because it is commonly believed that fatty acid utilization most often occurs after a minimum of 30 minutes of aerobic exercise. HIIT is somewhat counterintuitive in this regard, since most sessions are shorter than 30 minutes, but has nevertheless proven to burn fat even more effectively than long workouts. There are several factors that contribute to this, including the extended increase in RMR. HIIT also appreciably lowers insulin resistance and leads to skeletal muscle adaptations that result in improved glucose tolerance and enhanced skeletal muscle fat oxidation.

Recently it has been demonstrated that just two weeks of HIIT can considerably improve insulin action. "HIIT three times per week for 15 weeks compared to the same regularity of steady state exercise (SSE) provided substantial reductions in total body fat, subcutaneous leg and trunk fat, and insulin resistance. HIIT may then represent a feasible process for prevention of type-2 diabetes."

Cardiovascular disease:

A 2011 study by Buchan et al. evaluating the effect of HIIT on cardiovascular disease markers in adolescents reported that "brief, intense exercise is a time efficient means for improving CVD risk factors in adolescents".

For your cardio workouts, HIIT is recommended. It is effective and takes less time than traditional cardio training. You can incorporate simple 20 second on, 10 second off high intensity cardio into your exercise regimen or look for any HIIT routine that suits you. One example of a good HIIT workout that is simple to start with is to sprint or cycle as fast as you can for 20 seconds and walk or pedal slowly for ten seconds. Do this for at least 8 cycles for a quick workout. Be sure to stretch and warm up first and do some cool down activity after to avoid strain injuries. (Tip: Generally, if you can do HIIT for longer than 30 minutes before you're "worn out", you're not working intensely enough.)

If you choose HIIT for your cardio workout, pay attention to your heart rate just as in traditional cardio. For optimum benefits and fat loss your target heart rate (HR) should be within at least 20 beats per minute (BPM) of your maximum HR (but never over). For example, if you are 20 years old, your Max HR will be 200 and your goal should be to reach at least 180 bpm, but less than 200 bpm (180-199) when you are performing HIIT.

Here's how to calculate your max HR: Subtract your age from 220. For example, if you are 37, your max HR will be 220 - 37 = 183 bpm.

You should always consult your doctor before attempting to push your heart rate this high, especially if you have a pre-existing medical condition or are over 60 years old. The method above gives you a good estimate and your doctor can advise you on how to modify it to set a maximum heart rate that is healthy for you as an individual. Also, you will usually be advised to start at about 85% of this number if you aren't already used to high intensity cardio.[2]

---

[2] HIIT Reference: http://bit.ly/14Y7J32

Sample HIIT Routine:

## HIIT FAT BLASTING WORKOUT
Perform each exercise for 1 minute then rest for 30 seconds. Repeat 10 rounds

*Jump Rope
*Switch Jumps
*Burpees
*Pushups
*Plank Knee Tuck
*Jump Rope
*Kettle Bell Swings
*Twister Abs
*Burpees
*Lower Leg Raise
*High Knees
*Jump Rope
*Squat Twist
*Plank V-Up

Note: This workout should be 30 minutes.

    You can replace the jump rope parts with any type of cardiovascular exercise such as sprinting, cycling, fast swimming, etc. or even pretend to have a jump rope like I do. Just remember to adjust your intervals depending on the type of cardio you choose (for example, most people can't sprint for 60 seconds 10 times even with 30 seconds of rest in between). Make it work for you!

## Chapter 9: Keeping it Flat by Not Working Flat

Everyone eventually reaches a weight loss plateau. You will notice that your weight loss will eventually decrease and stop after a certain amount of time. There are simple methods you can use to avoid "going flat" in your quest to achieve flat abs.

Don't lower your caloric intake too much. It takes calories to burn calories. If you take in too few calories your body will just respond by lowering your metabolic rate, making it harder to lose weight. A good target for calorie reduction is within the 500-700 a day range. If you need to lose more calories, exercise.

Lean body tissue burns five times the calories than stored fat does. So keep those strength training workouts going to build lean body mass. Also keep up proper nutrition to support lean tissue growth and repair.

Losing weight itself will cause your BMR to go down. The less you weigh, the fewer calories you need to stay alive. Increasing lean body mass and supercharging your workouts as you build strength and endurance are sure ways to beat this.

Change your workout schedule and intensity. Varying the intensity and type of activity, as well as the time of day you do it keeps your body adapting and will not allow it to get used to your workout and hit a plateau. As you build more endurance, add more time to your HIIT (High Intensity Interval Training) workouts and as you build strength you may want to opt for heavier weights or more reps or sets.

Don't over-train. If you work out too much you will reach a point of diminishing returns. Your body will adapt to these overly physically stressful workouts and not burn as many calories and not put on as much lean mass as before.

Stick to these guidelines to keep yourself on track and your goal achievable! My blog also talks about this very topic; it's so important so please go ahead and check it out here: http://bit.ly/W4xo88.

The next chapter is on motivation and the chapters that follow provide greater detail on aspects of your new life such as proper diet, advanced exercises and cardio workouts and special training regimens for postpartum mothers, teenagers, etc.

## Chapter 10: Keeping it Fresh

Recall that I told you earlier that you have abs just like anyone else and that they are already in pretty good shape? Abs, like other core muscles are used every day in everything we do. That means that they get exercised all day, every day. They may not be "ripped" or "popping out" but they are definitely more toned than most other muscles in your body and in better shape overall. In fact, believe it or not, most body builders don't even work their abs directly. Some might do crunches once a week to pump them for a competition, but the abs are a major core muscle group and are thus exercised indirectly by properly executing exercises for other muscle groups. As an example, when doing bench presses in proper form, keeping your core engaged, (see above) your abs are being worked indirectly. So, all the targeted ab exercises in the previous chapter, even done for 10-20 minutes every other day are sure to get your abs just the way you want them.

This chapter is all about motivation and one major aspect of staying motivated is not to get bored. All the recommended workouts given in the previous chapters are proven to be effective and you have many different exercises to choose from for the strength training parts of your workout regimen. Still, there are many more great exercises out there and you should also feel the motivation to search and find good exercises that you find enjoyable. If you are keeping your journal properly you may have noticed that some exercises benefit you more than others. Everyone is unique and you need to find a good set of exercises that work well for you as an individual. I say "set of exercises" because doing the same exercise for too long leads to a plateau (and boredom). I always say, "Change up the reps and sets maybe add weight or take weight off." Keep on the lookout for new and unique ways to work out and look at your notes to find the moves that help you the best. Build a new workout routine from these as you go along and cycle through them to keep things fresh.

You actually have a head start as far as motivation is concerned. Your abs are already there and are getting better looking and stronger every single time you do strength training. Thus one major motivating factor for you to keep working out, sticking to your plan, is not to waste the abs you already have by allowing them to remain hidden by abdominal fat. Keep the cardio up so that all the work you've done sculpting your abs can be seen by the world--and you!

Remember what I mentioned in an earlier chapter, that you need to start enjoying the journey rather than wait and enjoy the end result. Enjoying the journey is lifelong enjoyment and the end result is basically one day of enjoyment. Many of you may ask, "How do I enjoy working out and doing tiring cardio; how do I enjoy the burn and the pain?" This is a valid question and the answer may surprise you.

While there are ways to make workouts more enjoyable, such as listening to music, varying routines, exercising with someone you find cute, etc. the truth is that very few people find enjoyment from the physical strain of exercising itself. What you need to focus on is the enjoyment you get from immediate satisfaction. Now, if you focus only on your goal of losing 40 pounds and revealing that six pack after 8 months or a year, you're going to be waiting for enjoyment for a long time. However, instant gratification is a powerful motivator in all of us. Thus, the key to remaining motivated, continuous enjoyment and to sticking to your plan is to provide yourself with instant gratification. Now your question is, "How do I do that?"

Ask yourself what your motivation is for getting fierce abs and how much a set of fierce abs really means to you. If you're a model, your motivation is to keep your job and keep doing what you love doing, and that super lean and tight tummy means a whole lot to you. But for most readers of this book this is not the case. Will achieving fierce abs make you a better parent or a kinder and more generous person? I wouldn't bet on it. Most of us are busy people with packed, stressful lives that will find it challenging enough just to incorporate the time for a workout plan into our daily schedules. So for all of us average people, the trick is to make our goals meaningful and functional and make sure that we get instant gratification from even one healthy meal or one hour of our regular workout. We have to change focus.

Take weight loss, fat loss and building a six pack off the table for now. Forget for the time being that these are the end goals and focus on immediate goals. Focus on your next meal and next exercise set and think about the following things. Exercise, both cardio and strength training, and proper nutrition does several things for us. Two immediate effects are: Energy to get through the next rough day and relief from tension and stress. If you take the focus off how much more fat you have to burn to reveal your abs and turn it to how much more energy you'll have to put into work and family today as well as anticipate the reduction in your stress level, you now have meaningful and functional goals. You now have your motivation for the day: Do your upper body workout to give you a boost of energy to get breakfast prepared and the kids off to school and get your cardio by walking to work, keeping the energy levels up and going as you work your day. Stay active in the office. Take the stairs up to the fifth floor every time you have to deliver a pile of papers to your boss. Do seated ab exercises while you're at your desk. Eat that healthy meal you packed which provides you with energy and nutrition but no guilt. Your energy level will keep up with your activity and nutrition level through the day and your instant gratification will be apparent when you get home and write in your journal that you didn't feel like falling asleep at your workstation today and you got good doses of vitamins A, B and C and minerals X, Y and Z from your meal at the office. You got home and fixed a healthy dinner for you and your family, spent quality time with them, alert and active, and your calorie balance for the day is -500. A few other benefits of enjoying life day to day like this are listed below--and there are many more.

- Being able to sleep more soundly and wake up feeling rested (Please read my article on why sleeping helps you get stronger - http://bit.ly/14i2dbb).
- Doing a great job at work every day. This will be noticed.
- Knowing you've accomplished something today and not a year from now.
- You're doing things every day that are keeping your body strong and healthy as you get older.
- No more anxiety from "I will start tomorrow". You're living it every day!
- You are being a good role model and nutritional provider for your family and friends.

As you lay in bed after your fierce day you think; you've had a great day. You felt great and still feel great. You're in an elevated mood and can't wait for tomorrow's fix-- and tomorrow's just around the corner. Now, some play time...

## Chapter 11: The Best, the Good, the Bad and the Ugly

In this chapter you will find the healthiest foods to eat and ingredients to cook with as well as the ones you really should avoid. First is a top ten list of healthy foods, then one of foods to avoid and following are the same for drinks.

### Top 10 Healthy Foods:

Almonds

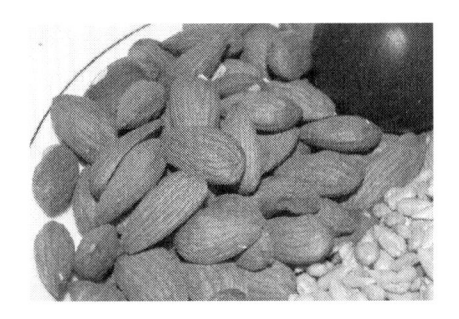

These tasty nuts contain hunger-satisfying protein and fiber. They have vitamin E, a potent antioxidant. They are also a great source of magnesium; this is a metal (mineral) that your body needs so it can burn calories, build new and repair existing muscle tissue, and regulate blood sugar levels. Stable blood sugar levels assist in staving off cravings that will cause overeating, and we all know that makes us gain weight. What makes almonds really fascinating (and cool) is their ability to "obstruct calories". Research shows that the makeup of the nut's cell walls may help to lessen the assimilation of the fat content of the cells in the nut--therefore, making them a very lean nut.

Eat about an ounce a day (that's about 23 almonds). This yields about 160 calories but even a handful of almonds can be very filling. (Tip: An Altoids tin will hold this amount perfectly.)

Eggs

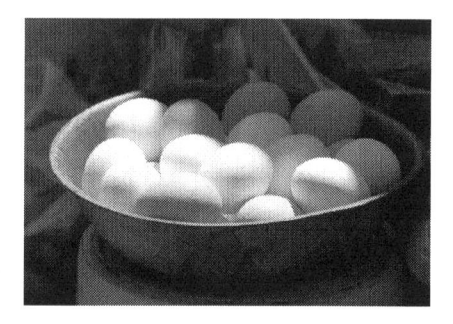

Eggs are considered the ideal protein source. Dietitians love and respect eggs because they have an amazing balance of essential amino acids (the building blocks of protein used by your body to produce everything from muscle fibers to neurotransmitters in the brain; and essential amino acids are those that your body cannot make by itself no matter what you eat so they have to come from a certain food itself--like eggs!). Researchers found that having eggs for breakfast made people feel less hungry the rest of the day compared to when they ate a breakfast of complex carbohydrates such as those found in bagels and breads (even the healthy whole grain kind).

One egg a day is healthy, best at breakfast, unless you have high bad cholesterol levels in your blood, in which case you should consult your family doctor about how often you can eat eggs. One large boiled egg has about 77 calories (60 in the yolk) and contains about 213 milligrams of cholesterol. A fried egg will yield about 89 calories.

Soy

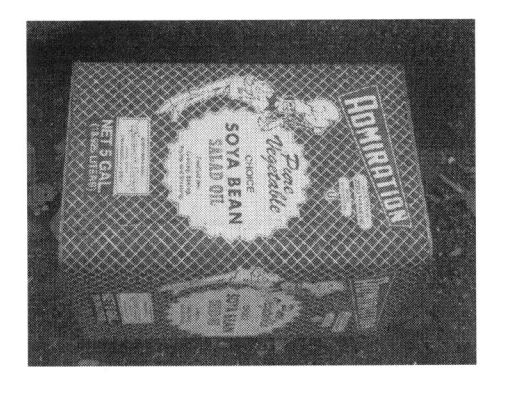

Soybeans contain a lot of antioxidants, fiber, and protein. They are also amazingly multipurpose. You can snack on roasted soybeans like nuts (dry-roasted, please), put shelled edamame into your soup, and use tofu as an ingredient in your healthy smoothie (a spoonful is good). Soy milk (or other liquid soy drinks) can also be used as a healthy meal replacement. In studies, overweight candidates who drank a soy milk-based meal replacement lost more weight than the subjects who drank a conventional dairy-based diet drink.

You should aim for about twenty-five grams of soy protein daily (whole soy protein, not isolated; the label should tell you). Four ounces of tofu yields about 94 calories and will give you about 10 grams of protein. Half a cup of edamame (steamed) yields about 130 calories and will give you about 11 grams of protein. Consume whole soy foods and not those with "isolated soy protein" as this may not supply all the health benefits of products made from whole soybeans.

Apples

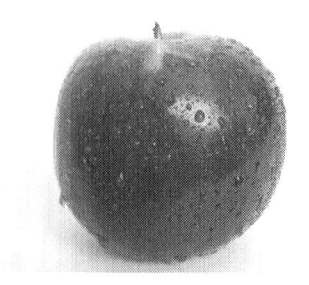

A 2003 study published in the journal *Nutrition* showed that overweight women in the group who incorporated three apples (or pears) each day into their nutrition plan for a three month period lost more weight than the women in the other group who were on a similar diet, but ate oat cookies rather than apples or pears. One large apple contains 5 grams of fiber, but it's also composed of almost 85 percent water; besides being essential for your body, water also helps you feel sated. Apples have a chemical in them called quercetin, which has been shown to help combat some types of cancer, reduce damage from high cholesterol, and support healthy lungs.

Incorporate a couple of apples a day into your diet. A study published in the *Journal of Agricultural and Food Chemistry* found that the following three varieties of apple had the highest antioxidant activity: Red Delicious, Cortland, and Northern Spy. The average, medium sized apple yields about 95 calories.

Berries

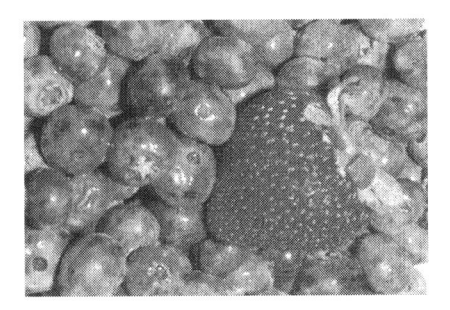

Most berries are very high in fiber--the "dieter's best friend". Experts say that the more fiber you eat the less fat you put on and the more you lose. They recommend an optimal dose of between 25 and 35 grams of fiber every day. Fiber prevents calories from being absorbed from all the other stuff you eat and drink. That's because fiber encloses food particles and carries them out of your digestive tract before they've been fully digested and macronutrients like fat and carbs have been fully absorbed. Berries, as well as other fruits, are also a very good source of antioxidants; these good chemicals help you get better outcomes from your workouts and have been shown to also help protect you from terrible diseases like cancer. Antioxidants work to improve blood circulation and this helps your muscles contract more resourcefully.

Consume at least one half cup of berries every day (this is about 30 calories). Don't just go for the most common ones, like raspberries, blueberries, and strawberries. Be adventurous, search for boysenberries, gooseberries, and black currants and add them to your mix for more variety in flavor as well as nutrition.

## Leafy Greens

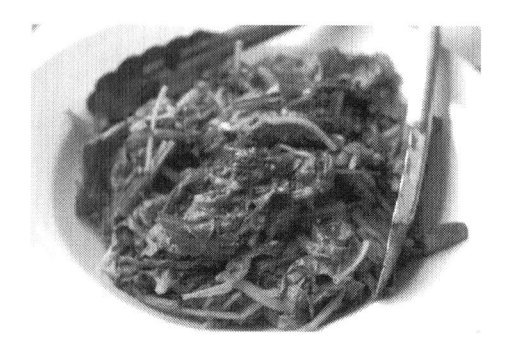

Cancer-preventing carotenoids in green, leafy veggies alone won't help slim your waist, but their ability to make you feel full while only giving you a few calories surely will. One cup of each of the following veggies only contains the number of calories given and gives you 20 percent of your daily fiber requirement: spinach, forty calories; broccoli, 55 calories... Most leafy greens also contain high levels of calcium, absolutely needed for muscle contraction during daily activity and workouts.

Three servings daily, one with each meal is recommended. (Tip: Have a ready bag of baby spinach, washed and ready to eat, in your fridge and throw a handful into almost everything you eat--not just salads-- such as: pasta dishes, sandwiches, soups and stir-fries.) Others that are just as good are kale (good for belly fat burning) arugula, broccoli, green beans or asparagus.

Lean Meats

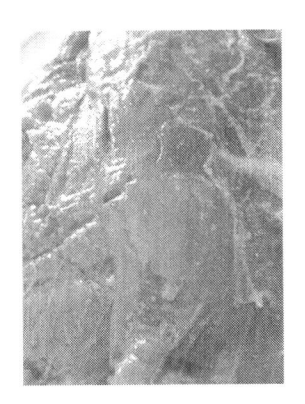

Chicken, Turkey (breast meat without skin is the leanest), lean or extra lean ground or white turkey meat are your best choices. The leanest cuts of red meat (but NOT pre-made or marinated) are also good as you have to vary your animal protein sources. Lean cuts of beef are: Arm Roasts, Bottom Round Steaks, Chuck Shoulder Roasts, Eye Of Round, Leg Cuts, Round Tips, Tenderloin Steak, Top Loin, Top Round Steaks, Top Sirloin and 90% Lean Ground Beef. Lean Pork cuts are: Bone-In Rib Chop, Bone-In Sirloin Roast, Bone-In Sirloin Roast, Boneless Top Loin Chop, Boneless Top Loin Roast, Center Loin, Ham, Pork Tenderloin and 90% Lean Ground Pork.

Bison is a very healthy option for a red meat. If you're ready to widen your meat horizons bison (commonly called American buffalo) is even lower in fat and calories than skinless light meat chicken! Deer and elk are nearly just as good for you if you have access to these wild meats. To compare, bison has only 2 grams of fat and 122 calories for a 3-ounce slice and. skinless chicken light meat chicken has 3 grams of fat and yields 144 calories. Bison is also a great source of protein; you get 24 grams for that three ounce serving and it also contains iron. It is comparable to beef in flavor, but with a slightly sweeter and richer flavor.

If you like lamb, get cuts from the shank half of the leg (ask the butcher if the label isn't clear). Shank-half cuts that have had the fat well-trimmed only have about 5 grams fat and 155 calories per serving.

Veggie Soup

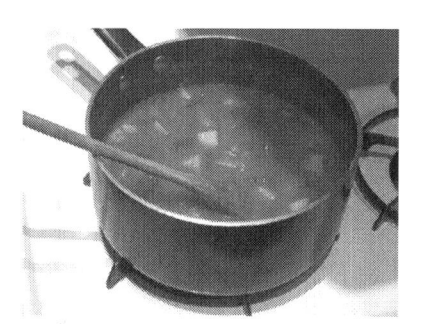

Researchers at Pennsylvania State University learned that eating broth-based (or low-fat cream-based) soups two or three times a day led to more successful weight loss compared to people who ate equal calories of various snack foods. Those who had a lot of healthy soup ion their diet also kept a total weight loss of 16 pounds after a one year observation period, on average. It's also a great way to vary your green vegetable intake.

Add at least one cup of veggie soup that is both low-calorie and low-sodium to your diet every day.

Salmon

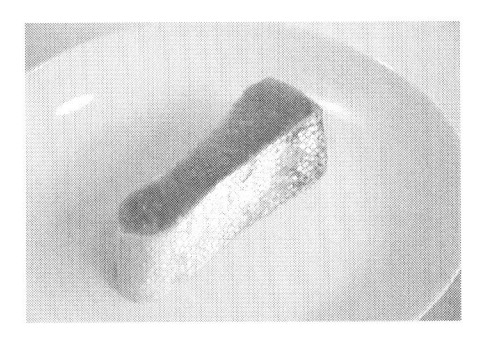

Salmon, tuna, and mackerel ("fatty fish") are excellent sources of omega-3 fatty acids. These super-healthy fats may help encourage fat burning by raising the efficiency level of your metabolism. An Australian study showed that overweight people who had fatty fish in their diet every day enhanced their glucose-insulin response. This means that fatty fish may help retard digestion and thus stave off cravings right after eating a full meal--a disastrous caloric addition. Additionally, these meats are excellent lean sources of protein for your ab regimen.

Two four-ounce servings each week is recommended. Wild salmon, though more expensive than farm-raised, has higher levels of omega-3 fatty acids. If the label doesn't say "wild", it's farm-raised.) If you don't like seafood, you can still get omega-3's from flaxseeds (pulverize well and add to your cereal). Walnuts are also high in omega-3's.

## Quinoa

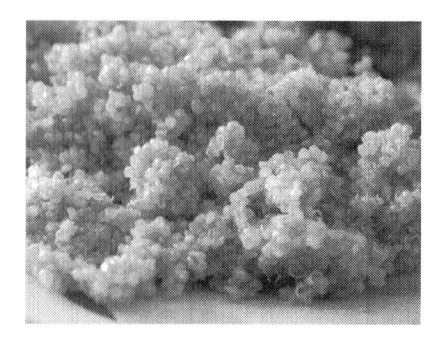

Pronounce it as KEEN-wah. This is a whole grain that has 5 grams of fiber and 11 grams of protein for every 1/2 cup serving. Prepare it just like any other grain (rinse if necessary). Quinoa has a nice, nutty flavor and a crunchy/chewy texture; it is sort of like a combination of whole wheat couscous and short-grain brown rice.

The recommended serving per day is at least one half-cup (this would be about 1/3 of your daily whole-grain needs). Try substituting AltiPlano Gold brand, which yields an average of 185 calories per packet), for your usual hot oatmeal servings. It can be found in health-food stores and comes in Chai Almond and Spiced Apple Raisin flavors.

## Almond Butter

In place of dairy, which is no good for abs, replace yogurt with almond butter. One tablespoon has 101 calories. It is high in good fats and low in bad fats (see below) and has no cholesterol. It contains dietary fiber, calcium and iron and has 2.4 grams of protein per 1 Tbsp. serving.

## Top 10 Foods to Avoid:

## Chips

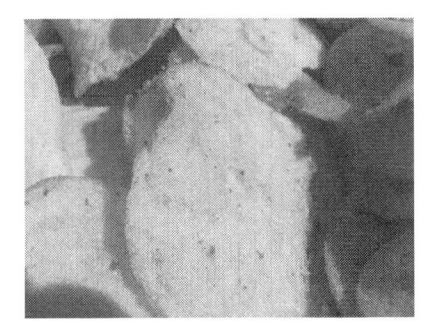

Just one ounce of potato chips will fill you with 152 calories and 10 grams of fat (three grams of which are saturated) and a small bag has over two ounces! If you eat just one and a half little bags a week, you'll have consumed over 23,400 calories and gained about seven pounds (most likely around your waist) in just one year. And most people eat over five times this amount or more. That's at least 117,000 calories and 35 pounds a year, every year! To put that into perspective, a 180 pound person would have to run 180 miles at 5 miles per hour just to burn all those calories off. Depending on your weight that would mean running a half mile every single day for a year--and that's just burning "chip calories", nothing else! What to eat instead: Rice and popcorn cakes have become tastier and more attractive to the palette now; they aren't styrofoam-like food anymore. They come in various flavors now and will satisfy your salty-crunchy cravings. Popular brands have less than 100 calories per serving. Edamame, when dry-roasted, is even better, 30 grams providing 14 grams of protein and one fifth (20%) of your iron requirement per day--all this for just 140 calories.

**Doughnuts**

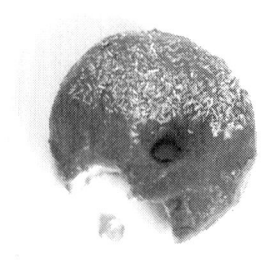

They are made of white flour and vegetable shortening--and they're probably deep-fried too--in bad fat. Here are some examples to scare you away from these holy things: A glazed Krispy Kreme (just one) yields 200 calories and 12 grams of fat, (and this includes a lot of saturated fat, Trans fat and cholesterol). An traditional cake doughnut contains 150% more calories than one Krispy Kreme as well as 28 grams of carbohydrates (the bad kind) and a killer 19 grams of fat (with 5 grams of it being saturated fat and 4 grams being trans-fat; almost half the fat content is nasty, really bad, heart-killing fat!). The American Heart Association recommends that a maximum of 30% of our calories should come from fat. That's would be around 65 grams for a 2,000-calorie daily a day diet; and if you're on a weight loss nutrition plan, you should keep it well below 30%.

What to eat instead: Eat whole-grain bagels to keep down the carbs. Half of a Pepperidge Farm multi-grain bagel has just 3 grams of fat, 125 calories and almost 4 grams of fiber to lower your cholesterol.

## Sausages

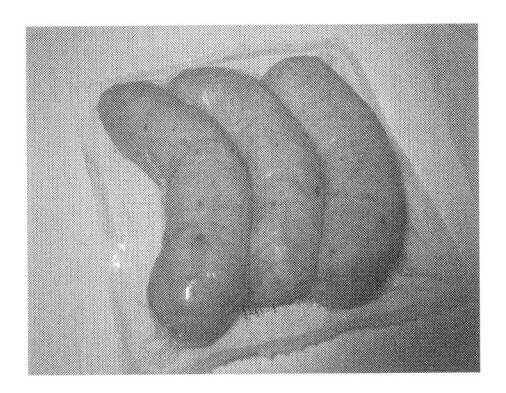

Even if you don't fry your sausages, most are an unhealthy food choice. One single pork link yields 217 calories and almost 20 grams of fat--just one short, unsatisfying link!

What to eat instead: Try chicken or turkey sausage, they are good substitutes. Five links of Aidell's chicken apple sausage have only 100 calories and 8 grams of fat, only 2.5 of which are saturated. Consider that you can eat over ten links of chicken sausage for every 1 link of pork sausage and the vast health difference becomes very clear...You can also go the vegetarian way: Boca Italian sausage (made from soy protein) has only 130 calories for a 2.5-ounce serving and just 6 grams of fat; but it gives you 13 grams of healthy, lean protein.

### Fried Chicken

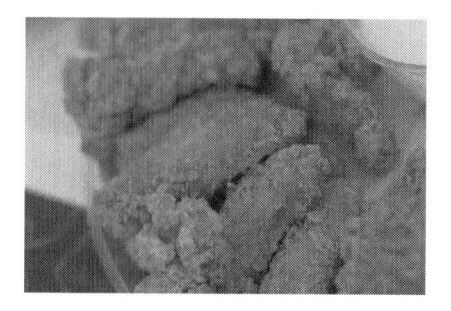

Chicken breast is a good healthy protein source, but when battered and fried packs nearly 400 calories and 22 grams of fat per serving. What to eat instead: Grilled, skinless chicken breasts are great if you prepare them right. Use a sizzling spice mix rub or try a green chili-lime marinade and barbecue them on a grill. You'll get a really nice flavor for just 189 calories per 4-ounce breast, plus the benefits of the pepper and hot spice you put on them!

### French Fries

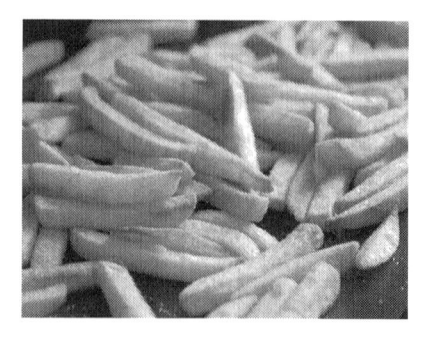

One large, 6 ounce order of fries from a typical fast food restaurant has about 570 calories--half of them are from fat! If you're having a burger with those fries (such as

Burger King's Whopper), add another 670 calories to the tally (and another 39 grams of fat)--A whopping 1240 calories and over 70 grams of fat from one meal! Consider this: A woman of average height with a reasonable target weight will probably have to limit her caloric intake to about 1500 calories a day. Add a drink to this meal and you're near that limit. Can you really be hunger-satisfied, and more importantly, will your body be getting proper nutrition from one burger meal a day? I say No Way!

What to eat instead:

If you MUST eat fries, ask for a smaller serving of fries instead like the kiddy size ("only" 230 calories and 13 grams of fat). At home, cook up some sautéed tempeh (this is a mixture of fermented rice and soy) you can find tempeh the refrigerated health-food section of your grocery store. Cut up the tempeh into fry-sized fingers, drizzle with a little soy sauce, and sauté in a tablespoon of olive oil (a healthy oil) until brown. Half a cup yields only 197 calories. Plus, unlike fries that are just starch and fat, tempeh is full of lean protein and is a good source of the following minerals: iron, zinc and magnesium; and it also contains vitamin B6, one of the three "B-complex" vitamins, which are essential daily nutrients for your nervous system among many other things.

## Soft White Bread and Processed Foods

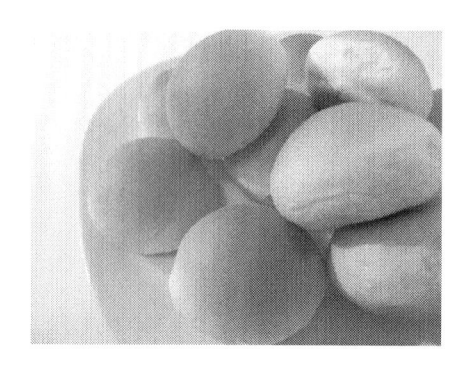

...are just as healthy for you as a candy bar. One slice of white bread offers you little more than 65 calories from white flour, a non-complex and quickly digested carbohydrate; these "bad" carbs will cause your blood sugar to spike and then crash--this is what simple sugars do. Bread and pastries made from processed-to-death white flour have so few nutrients that your hunger will return quickly soon after eating because you will crave the fiber and vitamins your body is looking for from a meal.

What to eat instead: A slice of whole-wheat bread has a nice nutty flavor, 2 grams of fiber, protein, and nutrients like selenium, magnesium and potassium for the same number of calories. Also eat whole grain bagels, English muffins, scones, and muffins instead. Their fiber content will fills you up so you will eat less but feel satisfied. But make sure they are all whole grain or wheat! No white flour bagels or muffins allowed.

## ALSO AVOID:

### Fried Wontons

These triangular snacks or appetizers are filled with meat or shrimp (and now, even cream cheese!) and they are deep-fried to make them crispy and crunchy, the deep frying adding tons of unhealthy oil and fats. These bite-size food items may seem harmless, but they can quickly add up to a whole meal's worth of calories-- without filling you up. A mere four crab and cream cheese-filled wontons contain 311 calories and 19 grams of fat.

What to eat instead: For some crunch, have some brown-rice sesame crackers; only 140 calories and 6 grams of fat for a five piece serving; this will also give you 1 gram of fiber and a large dose of calcium. They will satisfy your salty snack craving.

### Imitation Cheese in a Can

I don't know why some people love this stuff. There's plenty of way-better tasting healthy cheese out there. Two tablespoons (what you'd put on just two crackers) contains 276 calories and 21 grams of fat, 13 grams of which are saturated--for a lousy, unsatisfying, two cracker snack (and don't forget to add the calories and fat from the crackers)!

What to eat instead: Go for the real deal. Delicious soft cheeses such as brie have about 100 calories an ounce. Goat cheese is healthier still: An ounce serving yields just 76 calories plus 5 grams of protein.

## Non-Dairy Toppings

As delicious as they are, Cool Whip and similar products are mostly corn syrup and hydrogenated vegetable oil. You really don't want this stuff in your body, and it does tend to stay once taken in. Just one tablespoon yields 32 calories, but no one eats just one tablespoon...

What to eat instead: Top desserts with whipped egg white with just a little sugar. This is an excellent protein source and you will get protein while eating dessert! Home-made meringue with just a little sugar tastes just like artificial toppings and you won't have the bad stuff or the guilt.

## Fettuccine Alfredo

White flour pasta sopping with butter, cream and parmesan cheese. Thoroughly tasty, yes, but--a 3 ounce serving (only the size of a small woman's fist) packs 543 calories and 33 grams of fat (19 of them saturated). The average serving is about 8 ounces: 1148 calories and way more than your fat quota for a whole day just from one meal.

What to eat instead: Buy or ask for whole-wheat fettuccine and eat the pasta with marinara sauce. A cup of whole-wheat pasta contains just 197 calories plus about 4 grams of fiber. And 1/2 cup of marinara sauce yields only 92 calories. (Tip: If you can't order whole-wheat pasta, try asking for spinach pasta. It's more common than whole-wheat pasta and has a lot of nutrients, not just good carbs.

## **Best Healthy Drinks:**

Coconut Water

This drink is becoming a hot trend, and rightly so. Did you know that during World War II, raw, unprocessed coconut water was used as a direct replacement for intravenous drips for the injured, both soldiers and civilians? Pretty hard to believe, but look it up. Coconut water is so healthy and such the perfect drink for electrolyte balance that it can be used almost straight out of the coconut and direct into your bloodstream! Look it up, I'm sure you're dying to. It contains natural potassium, sodium and magnesium that are artificially added to sports drinks, and contains these electrolytes in near perfect balance. There's no other drink in the world like it. If you can't get whole coconuts and have to buy bottled or canned coconut water, be sure to read the label for any additives you don't want such as extra sugar or other processed additives.

Water

You've heard this before and you're going to hear it again. There is no substitute for plain water. Yes, I said coconut water was a miracle drink but ordinary water is still the best for you. In the US and other countries where tap water is purified there is no reason to spend money on pricey bottled water. Most bottled water comes from the municipal supply anyhow (not the top of Mt. Fuji)--read the label carefully. If you do buy bottled water, don't get the brands that put extra minerals in and definitely DO NOT drink distilled water. The magic of water is that you can control your electrolyte levels separately. Mineralized water may contain too many minerals, leading to dehydration and distilled water will leach precious minerals from your body. A chilled jug of water from your kitchen with a handful of mint leaves thrown in is an amazingly healthy and refreshing workout drink--as well as for the rest of the day. You want to aim for a gallon a day and break it up as best you can throughout your day.

### Low Sodium V8 Juice

V8 juice literally is Liquid Vegetables. It gives you good amounts of sodium and potassium plus all the benefits of real vegetables in a tasty drink. High in water content, drinking an 8 ounce glass before a workout will give you a healthy energy and nutritional boost. It's almost $4.00 for a 46 ounce bottle but you can always make your own. Read the label, buy the ingredients and blend away!

### **Drinks to Avoid:**

### Soda

Chock full of high fructose corn syrup, non-diet soda will overdose you with processed sugars that are high in calories and will give you a sugar crash. The combination of extreme sugar content and no other nutritional value makes you crave food and can lead to binge eating when you crash after drinking. Diet soda does not have sugar but the artificial sweeteners in it are also not healthy and studies have linked them to numerous diseases and conditions. Artificial sweeteners are known to make your body crave for real sugar.

### Fruit Juice From Concentrate and Fruit-Flavored Drinks

Concentrates may contain 20% actual juice but they have none of the fiber in natural juice and are loaded with processed sugars and high fructose corn syrup. Fruit-flavored drinks are even worse, most containing no real juice at all, just artificial flavors and, you guessed it, sugar. The amount of sugar in these drinks is so high that they can actually dehydrate you, making you crave for more, leading to a vicious cycle. There's just not enough water in them to excrete all the excess sugar they contain. They do contain small amounts of vitamins, but not enough to make them worth it. They are just a tiny bit better than soda, very tiny. If you have a juicer or a blender it really doesn't take much to make your own 100% fruit juice drinks.

## Sports and Energy Drinks

Sports drinks do contain electrolytes but they have too much sugar, making their water content inadequate to process everything that's in them. If you sweat for more than an hour and sweat profusely, you do need electrolyte replenishment but it is better to drink water and eat some fruit such as bananas and melons to get your electrolytes. The sugar in sports drinks is refined while fruit sugars are a bit more complex and won't lead to sugar crashes.

Energy drinks have energy-boosting ingredients, the most natural being caffeine. They have a lot more sugar than sports drinks and will give you both a caffeine and a sugar crash. Caffeine is a diuretic (it makes your body get rid of more water in your urine) and thus can dehydrate you. A typical energy drink, per volume, has four times the caffeine contained in a Coke. They also contain taurine and inositol which can upset your neurotransmitter balance in your brain. They can be addictive.

## Fancy Coffee

Coffee, hot or iced, topped with a ton of whipped cream, caramel, etc. such as a typical Starbucks order is full of simple sugars and fat. Coffee in itself is healthy for you taken in moderation but this refers to brewed coffee with sugar to taste, best made by yourself. Adding some milk or cream is not bad; just watch your portions and servings.

## Ethanol

This is the scientific name for the alcohol in hard liquor, wine and beer. Alcoholic beverages leach your body of huge amounts of water and B vitamins, both essential for energy production. Alcohol is also very high in calories. Typical calorie counts are as follows: One can of beer has about 210 calories; a glass of Bailey's Irish Cream has 140, a glass of wine, 90, and a shot of vodka, 55. And liquor has no nutritional value unless you count its sugar content. (Sugar is a macronutrient but this is not a good way to get it.)

Cocktails such as Pina Colada, Long Island Iced Tea, etc. also fall under this category because of their alcohol content but are even worse because of the added sugar. One Margarita can have up to 740 calories. That's one big meal. A virgin (alcohol-free) cocktail will generally have fewer calories but still around the 400-550 calorie mark. That's the same amount of calories in a small home-grilled burger made with very lean ground beef and low fat cheese and mayo.

Note that all these "bad" drinks can be consumed in moderation. It would be worse for your motivation if you had to look to a future of never touching these things again. The best path to take is to just watch the amounts you consume. If you've done an extra few hours of strength training and/or cardio in the last few days, go ahead and use one of these drinks as a reward. Remember, they are not deadly poisons. If you have a soft drink or a cocktail once in a while, it could be good for morale. Just get out of the habit of substituting things like energy drinks and soda for water if you're thirsty. One great rule to follow is that if you're thirsty or have a craving for one of these drinks, have a glass or two of water (or any other healthy drink) first and then, being sated, sip on your Red Bull like it was a glass of champagne and enjoy it. I really do mean that.

The next section breaks down food sources into three main groups: Protein, Carbohydrates and Fats. Lists are given for the best and worst sources of each.

## Top 17 Sources of Protein:

Note: Many of the best sources of protein listed are plant protein sources. They are considered the best sources because they have low or no fat and cholesterol and are high in fiber and also provide vitamins and minerals. The drawback of plant sources is that most are low in protein. If you do not supplement plant protein with animal protein from the healthy sources listed you will have to consume more calories to get your daily protein requirement. Most nutritionists recommend consuming animal protein since most plants do not contain all the essential amino acids (the ones our bodies cannot make themselves). One of the few plant sources of protein that contains all eight essential amino acids in one single food is Spirulina, however, to get the required amount of essential amino acids from Spirulina alone would require you to consume 5 grams of Spirulina powder (or capsules) a day and this is pricey. Furthermore, recent evidence from a complete study on the first generation of vegans and vegetarians who ate no animal protein showed that their lifespan was, on the average, ten years shorter than people who ate normal amounts of animal protein. think about that!

All the animal sources are relatively low in fat if you choose and prepare properly (such as cooking chicken and turkey without skin) and are complete proteins (have all eight essential amino acids). Read labels carefully and choose meat with less than 15% fat content and avoid meat with heavy marbling.

Make sure you get your required amount of protein per day. Here is the recommended way to calculate this:

1) Take your weight in pounds and divide that number by 2.2 (this is your weight in kilograms).

2) Multiply your weight in kg by 0.8-1.8 depending on your level of activity, health and condition (E.g. 0.8-0.99 if you are sedentary or exercise very little, have low stress levels and aren't pregnant or lactating and in good health and 1.0-1.8 if you are recovering from illness, exercise vigorously, are pregnant, under a lot of stress, etc. Also, males will need to use a slightly higher multiplier.) There are not enough studies to give exact multipliers for various individuals but use the example below to guide you.

Example: 154 lb. female in good health, lactating who does cardio and weight training 4-5 times a week
154 lbs. /2.2 = 70 kg
70 kg x 1.4 = 98 grams of protein/day

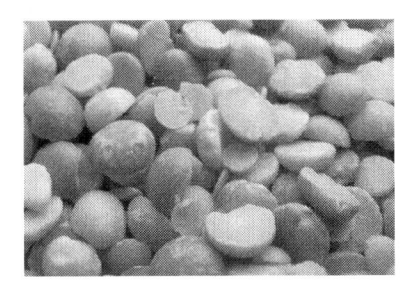

1. Lentils: They are high in protein and also provide you with fiber and minerals and micronutrients, such as iron and folate. 100 grams of lentils yields 23.2 grams of protein.

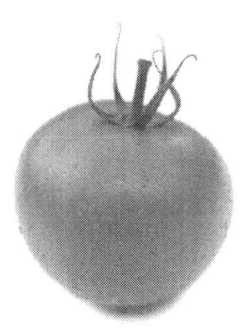

2. Tomatoes: Eating more fruits and vegetables will help prevent diseases and will make you feel full and satisfied without consuming huge amounts of calories. They have hardly any fat or calories and give you fiber and numerous key micronutrients. Tomatoes won't give you much protein, just 1 gram per fruit, but are a great overall diet supplement[3] so you'll need protein sources

---

[3] I've included them in the top sources of protein since you can eat several tomatoes and thus get several grams of protein without significant intake of calories and fat. For

in your diet that contain more protein per serving, especially if strength training with weights. You'll get the most protein per serving if you make your own pasta sauce from tomatoes and eat them that way, but remember to use whole-wheat or spinach noodles for "good" carbs and extra protein.

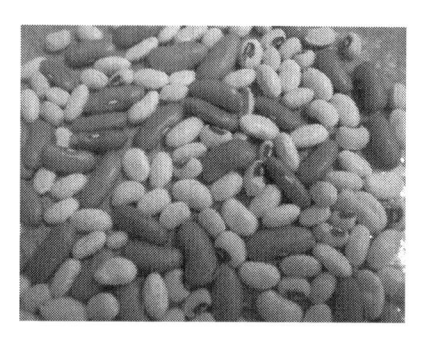

3. Beans: Beans provide you with protein, fiber and many important nutrients. Beans have an average of 8.5 grams of protein per cooked half cup.

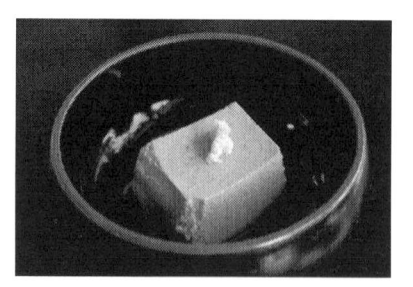

4. Tofu: An excellent source of plant protein. One half cup has 20 grams of protein.

---

example, if you made your pasta sauce from scratch, you'd get about 10 grams of protein from your pasta sauce alone. Not bad.

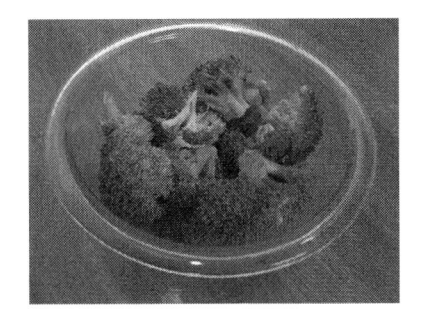

5. Broccoli: Broccoli provides only 2 grams of protein per one cup serving, so while it is very healthy and should be part of your diet, include food in your diet that is higher in protein content. Although the same rule applies as for tomatoes; you can eat a ton of broccoli if you really like it and get quite a lot of protein and very few calories and almost no fat.

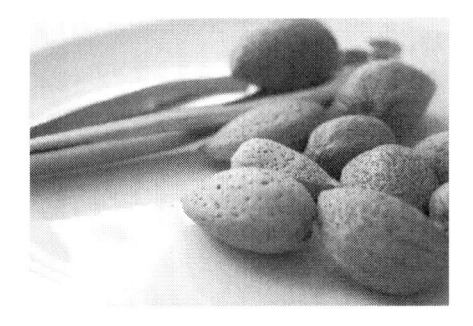

6. Nuts: These seeds are a great source of protein and healthy (monounsaturated) fats. One-fourth cup of nuts provides an average of 5.75 grams of protein. Peanuts and almonds provide 9 and 8 grams respectively and pecans, 2.5 grams. Choose low-sodium, dry-roasted nuts.

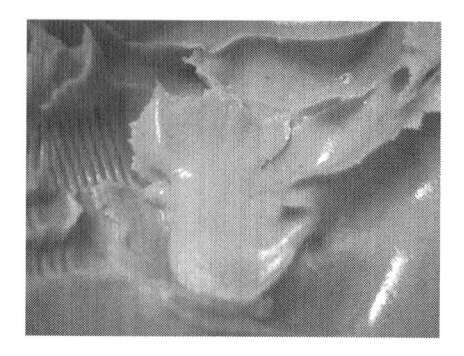

7. Peanut Butter: The peanut is a pretty amazing nut and peanut butter provides almost all the benefits of peanuts. Look for unsweetened peanut butter without added oil in the ingredients to avoid extra sugar and partially hydrogenated oils, both unhealthy. One tablespoon of peanut butter yields almost 4 grams of protein.

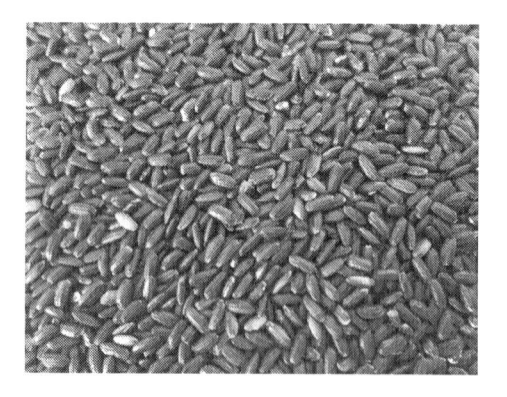

8. Rice: Choose unpolished brown rice. It is not processed and polished like white rice so it retains its fiber content as well as other nutrients (including plant protein). Whole grains, such as quinoa or millet are also healthy grains for your nutrition plan. Brown rice has about 5 grams of protein per cup.

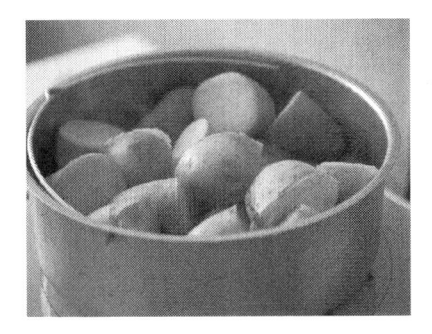

9. Potatoes: High in potassium and other vitamins and minerals, an average potato with skin yields about 5 grams of protein.

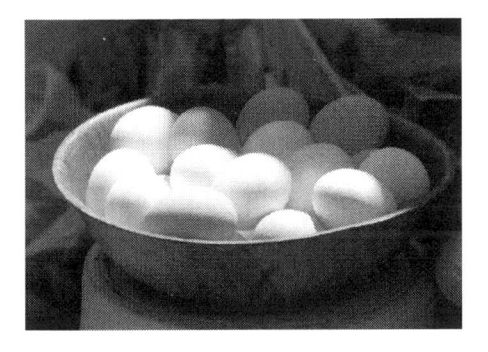

10. Eggs: One egg a day, at breakfast is best and recommended. One large egg provides 6 grams of protein.

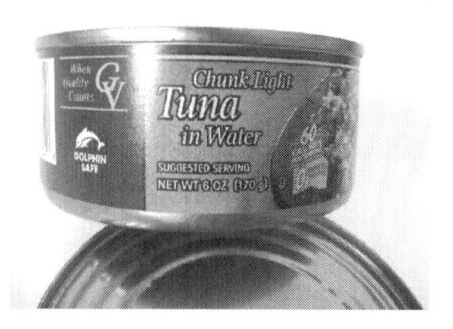

11. Tuna: Rich in Omega-3 fatty acids. Choose light tuna (and packed in water, not oil) to reduce mercury exposure. A 6 ounce can yields 40 grams of protein. Another good choice is Albacore Tuna.

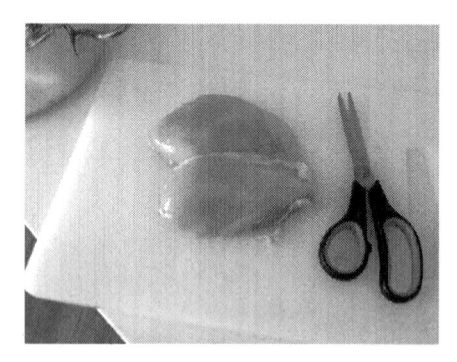

12. Chicken: This is the best meat to include in your nutrition plan. Cook it without the skin to minimize your intake of saturated fat. One 3.5 ounce breast provides 30 grams of protein.

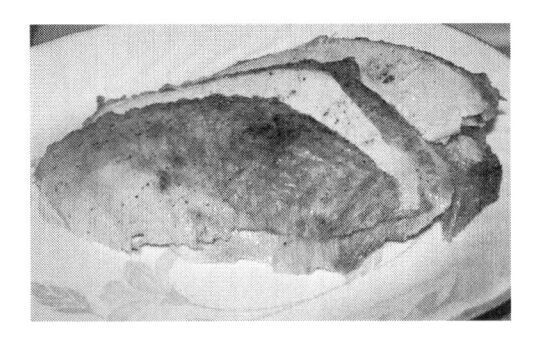

13. Turkey: Don't choose the processed forms (cold cuts, sausage, etc.); they aren't really healthy. A 3 ounce breast yields 22 grams of protein.

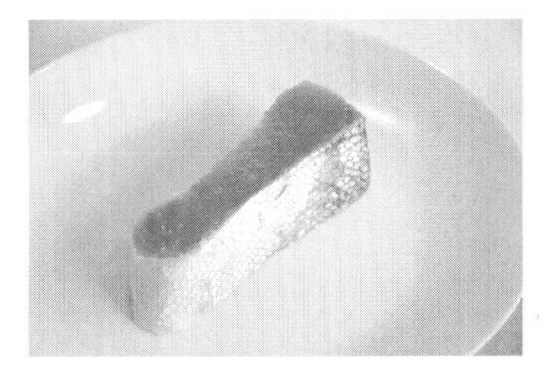

14. Salmon: Choose wild salmon over farmed, if you can get it for the highest amount of healthy omega-3 fatty acids. Eat salmon and other fatty fish like mackerel several times a week. A 3 ounce fillet gives 22 grams of protein.

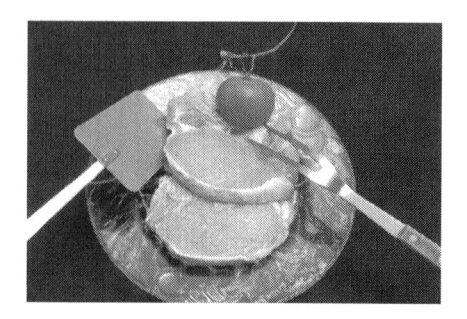

15. Pork: Skip processed pork, like bacon. One chop (about 5 ounces yields 33 grams of protein.

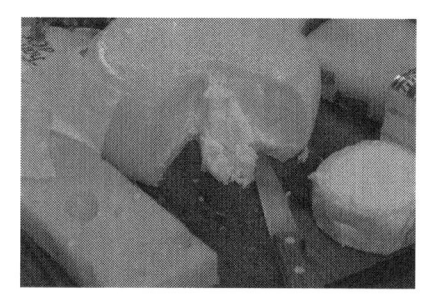

16. Cheese: Have a single serving (1.5 ounces for hard cheese) If you eat the sharply flavored hard cheeses you will get the maximum flavor impact for fewer calories and fat. Also, choose low-fat cheese, when possible. Part-skim mozzarella is good and so is low-fat cottage cheese. Cheese, on average gives you about 7 grams of protein per ounce. Hard cheeses like mozzarella and parmesan yield about 9.5 grams of protein per ounce but have more fat than soft cheeses such as cottage cheese at 5 grams per ounce.

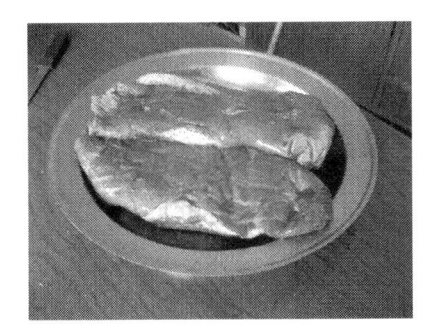

17. Beef: Look for grass-fed beef as the healthiest option. While pricier than grain-fed, it is richer in omega-3 fats--fats you want in your diet. Also avoid processed beef products, like sausage, since processing takes out nutrients and adds fat.

### **Top 10 Best Sources of Carbohydrates:**

**1. Oats**

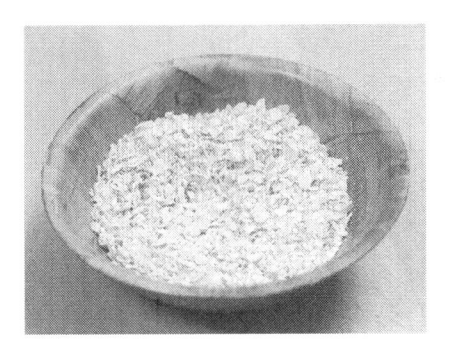

Buy some whole oats, grind them up (a coffee grinder is good for this) and put some in your protein shake. Or boil the oatmeal and top it with peanut butter for a tasty snack.

**2. Yams/Sweet Potatoes**

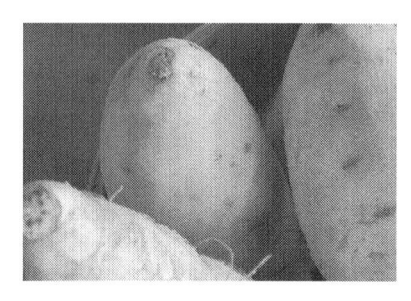

Stick them deep with a fork to prevent explosions, and cook them in the microwave for a few minutes for no fat-added and fast cooking. This is a ready to eat source of healthy carbs.

**3. Brown Rice**

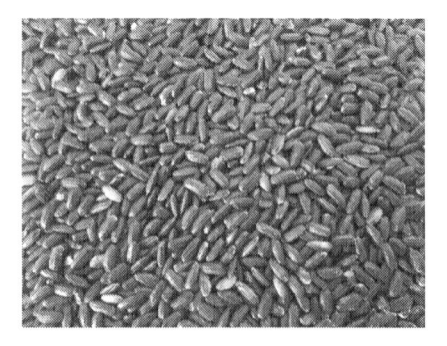

Brown rice takes a little more time to prepare. Use a rice cooker to simplify things. Rice cookers also keep the cooked rice warm for you.

## 4. Broccoli

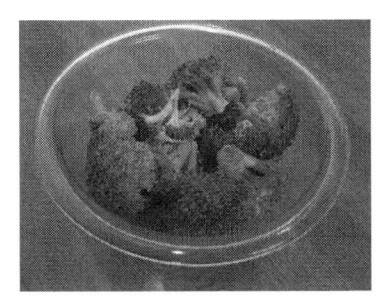

This can be eaten raw or cooked. Take a bag of raw mixed veggies with you and add some healthy crunch to your meals. Boiling broccoli is the best way to cook it although stir frying with olive oil is also healthy if you use a non-stick pan and just a tablespoon of oil. Eating vegetables raw preserves more nutrients than cooking them. Boiling them into a soup and consuming the liquid is the second best choice.

**5. Spinach**

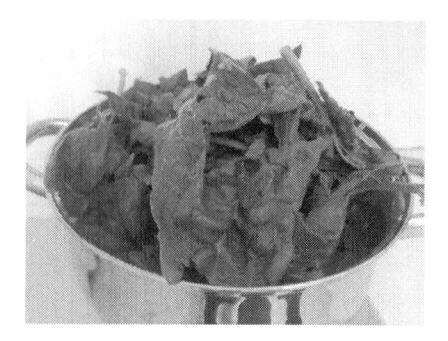

Take raw spinach and use some in your salads to enhance the nutritional value of your salad. Put some spinach in your breakfast omelet too.

**6. Peppers**

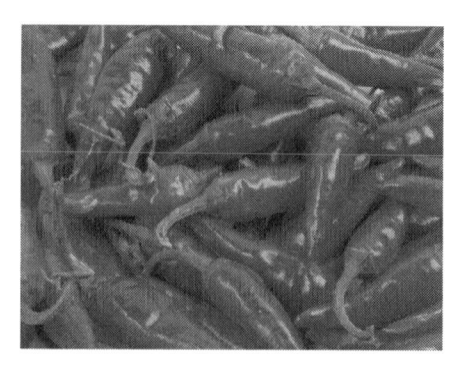

Chop some up and add them to your daily veggie bag. Any color you can find is fine; green, yellow, orange, red, they are all healthy. Peppers taste great and are healthiest raw. Peppers boost your metabolism and make you burn more calories even while resting. Adding them to soups gives you a filling, nutritious, low-calorie meal that revs up your metabolism. Now, a nutritious, filling, low-cal soup dish that makes you burn calories is a really magical meal!

**7. Beans**

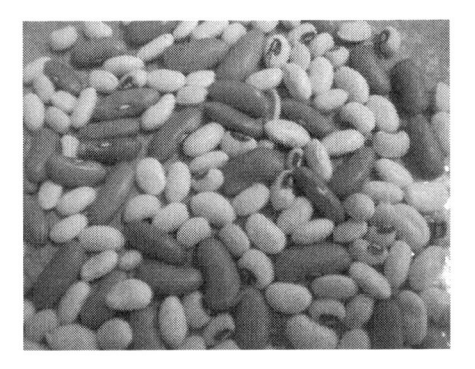

Mixing beans with your chili and tomatoes, tomato paste or sauce and lean ground or shredded beef makes a great meal. You can also add black beans to your brown rice serving. Beans also go well with lots of different foods and they contain a lot of protein.

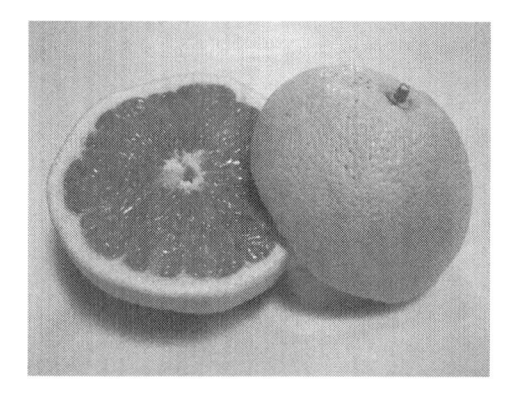

## 8. Grapefruit

Grapefruit has high fiber content and lots of vitamin C.

## 9. Berries

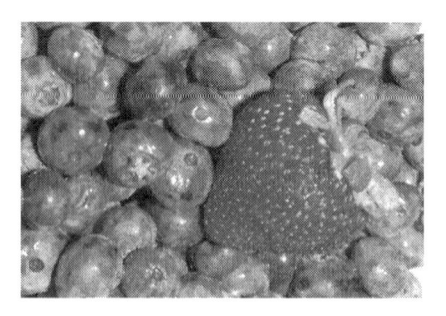

All berries are terrific sources of carbohydrates. They can be found in the freezer section of the grocery or can be bought fresh at the market. Make a protein shake in the blender and throw in several kinds of berries for a great workout shake.

**10. Apples**

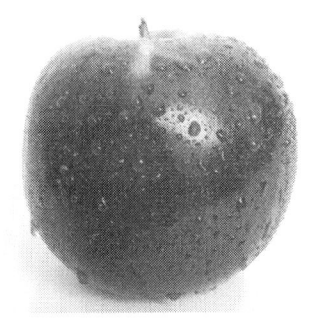

Studies show that eating 2-3 apples a day promotes weight loss. (NOTE: DO NOT peel the apple and throw away the peeling — that's where most of the vitamins and minerals are!

**Best Sources of Healthy Fats:**

Monounsaturated Fats:

- Canola oil
- Olive oil
- Sesame oil
- Sunflower oil
- Peanut oil
- Olives
- Avocados
- Peanut butter
- Nuts (peanuts, pecans, almonds, hazelnuts, cashews, macadamia nuts)

Polyunsaturated Fats:

- Safflower oil
- Soybean oil
- Corn oil
- Tofu
- Flaxseed
- Walnuts
- Soymilk
- Sunflower, pumpkin, and sesame seeds
- Fatty fish (tuna, salmon, herring, mackerel, sardines, trout)

## Chapter 12: The Must Have Grocery List

To sum up all the nutritious food items you should have in stock, here is a sample grocery list with the foods given above and some others that are great for your abs!

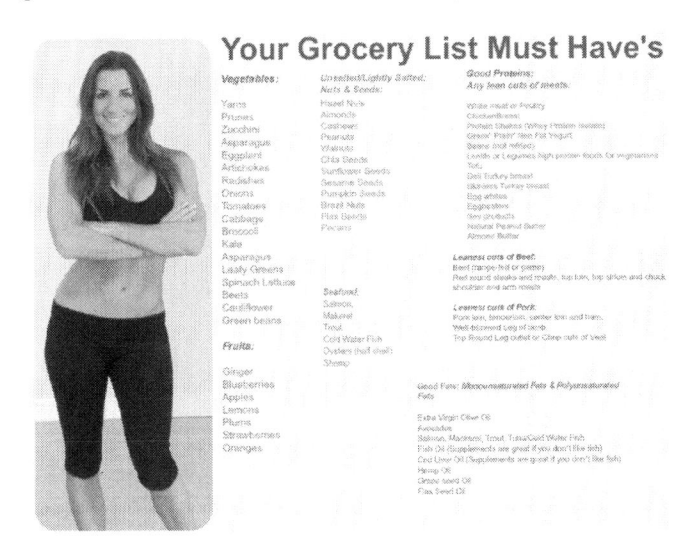

If you prefer to have a hard copy that you can download and print out go to http://bit.ly/XEO0PA and get your free copy now!

You should be able to plan a varied, tasty and healthy diet with the foods given above. You can find complete nutritional information for all of these foods online including things such as such as sugar content, sodium, etc. if you have any special concerns regarding any health conditions you may have.

## Chapter 13: Just Say "Na"[4]

"Na" is the chemical symbol for Sodium--and we generally should say No to sodium. Commonly known as salt, it is found naturally in most foods and performs an indispensable role in maintaining the best possible health and running of your body--in the proper amount, that is. The Dietary Guidelines for Americans established by the U.S. Departments of Agriculture and Health and Human Services recommend that no more than 2300 mg (2.3 grams) of sodium per day is what adult women should consume. Most women, though, consume more than this daily recommended allowance (over 2.7 grams) and this, of course, has negative consequences to their health. American men consume even more sodium, more than 4,000 mg sodium each day, and many people consume 7 grams without noticing. You do need a small amount, about 200 mg a day minimum, to stay alive and to keep fluids in balance. The Institute of Medicine recommend 1,500 milligrams (mg) of sodium per day, with a maximum dose of 2,300 mg (see above).

**Sodium and Health**

Sodium is a required element of your daily nutrition plan, and the Institute of Medicine advises that adults take in at least 1500 mg per day. Sodium aids your body in keeping the proper equilibrium of fluids, and it regulates your blood pressure and blood volume. Sodium helps your nerves send their electrical signals, and it also used in the actions of muscles (contraction and relaxation).
Your kidneys are the organs in your body that process

---

[4] Sodium Reference: http://bit.ly/WyjrxX

and store your optimum sodium equilibrium for your body's operation. They store sodium when your intake levels are not high enough, and they expel excess sodium through your urine when your intake and internal levels are too high.

Excessive Sodium Consumption strains your kidneys and impairs their functioning, which can lead to high blood pressure (hypertension). Because sodium makes your body retain water, extreme intake leads to higher blood volume which increases the work load on your heart to pump blood through your circulatory vessels. Hypertension is a known and major risk factor for stroke and heart ailments. Research from the American Heart Association shows that these are the two leading causes of death for Americans.

**High levels of sodium in the body also make you retain water, causing stomach bloating, which then hides your abs even if you're already trim.**

**Sources of Sodium**

Sodium in your diet normally comes from three major sources. The main sources are processed foods, such as TV dinners, canned soups, cold cuts and fast food (which have large amounts of added salt). Sodium is also found naturally in vegetables, dairy products, meat and shellfish; although these foods do contain less sodium than processed food and meals, but consuming too much natural sodium is still damaging to your health. The third main supply, which is easily avoided, is the salt in your kitchen or in the salt shaker on your table.

**Finding a Healthy Balance**

Like most Americans, you would do well to drop your intake. Experts at the Mayo Clinic advise that "you can lower your sodium intake by eating more fresh fruits and vegetables". If you add more potassium-rich foods to your nutrition plan, you can compensate for the harmful effects of sodium on hypertension. Foods rich in potassium include fruits that grow on vines and dark, leafy, green vegetables. To add rich flavor of your meals without using a lot of salt, use various tasty herbs, citrus peel and fresh squeezed fruit juice.

Note: These are provided as general recommendations. If you have hypertension or other medical conditions, consult your physician for the amount of sodium you need each day as an individual particular to the state of your health.

**Chapter 14: Bad Smoothie!**

Not all smoothies are created equal. Fast food smoothies are far from healthy. Even those that come from gyms, shops or stands that specialize in smoothies are usually loaded with sugar and sometimes fat.

Check this out: A Smoothie King's The Hulk-Strawberry (20-ounce serving) contains more calories than a Burger King Double Cheeseburger and a regular order of French fries (Total: 990 calories, 52 grams of fat--19 grams are saturated fat). Dairy Queen's Tropical Blizzard (1,122 calories, 62 grams total fat--25 grams of it saturated!) has more fat (including saturated fat) in it than the Burger King meal given above. Bad smoothies!

Let's face it; we have the wrong idea about what makes a "good smoothie." We have been lead to believe that just because we're substituting a meal with a smoothie that we will lose weight. The world today is full of fattening fast food masquerading as healthy food, and the smoothie is no different. Recent studies have shown that some smoothies commonly served in fast food restaurants have thousands of calories in them-- THOUSANDS! When you order a smoothie, you definitely might want to take a careful look at the ingredients list. If it comes with whipped cream, that is definitely not a healthy drink. If your smoothie has ice cream in it, or blended pieces of cookies or chocolate bits, it's not a healthy smoothie either.

Here is how to make or order a healthy smoothie: Smoothie recipes with yogurt are a good place to start, as you have all the helpful stomach bacteria of yogurt, as well as high calcium content for your muscles and bones. A healthy smoothie is one that is loaded with fruits--that's fruits, plural, so look for variety in the types of fruits in your smoothie. But keep in mind to keep fruit and yogurt low, they are not good for seeing Fierce Abs!

Sugar makes you fat and dairy is a no-no when trying to achieve abs. But as a general guideline you should have some fruits and yogurt in your nutrition plan. Just start to learn how to prepare your shakes to make them perfect for you!

Different combinations of fruits can have very different nutrient profiles. You don't want a smoothie, for example, that is getting most of its nutrition from ripe banana calories. True, bananas are great for you, but you want nutritional variety in your smoothies. Look for at least three ingredients in your smoothie, strawberry-peach-banana, for example. Be creative, mix colors and have a big slice of the rainbow inside your smoothie. This is an easy way to make sure that you are getting a lot of different types of the antioxidants in various fruits.

Now get even more creative. Add some unconventional items to it that you may not have considered before. Avocados are a great addition. Avocados contain a ton of very healthy fats and are one of the very best foods that you can eat, in moderation of course, just like anything else. Since avocados are so high in fat, they can really make a smoothie seem creamy tasting without having to add unhealthy fats to it. Almonds are another food that are really good for you, and great in smoothies. Almonds are very high in protein and have nutrients that are excellent for your brain health. Many neuroscientists consider almonds to be an underused brain food. Tests with mice prove it. Almonds help mice perform various tasks faster. Almonds may also be effective at delaying Alzheimer's. Studies show that almonds may help the brain in numerous other ways as well, such as improving memory. Best of all, almond butter really adds a rich buttery flavor to many smoothies.

If you like your smoothies a little lighter, try adding spinach leaves and kale; its sweet flavor will go well with most fruits. If you are really adventurous, try adding a veggie or two into your smoothie. It's not hard at all.

Another good way to add great nutritional benefit and make your smoothie super-healthy is to add a little fresh ginger to it. Ginger has a lot of great health benefits, such as powerful anti-inflammatory effects. Ginger has also been found to boost immunity and fight off cancer. Not bad for just adding a little spice to your smoothie, huh?

Watch those bad smoothies and don't be afraid to experiment with the myriad of healthy ingredients available out there. Always try to add whey protein powder for a recovery shake. A healthy smoothie will help you with weight loss & strengthen your immune system.

## Chapter 15: Fat Burners?

No. Here's why:

Most of the 'Fat Burners' for sale are just overpriced caffeine; they are basically artificially produced caffeine in elevated doses, mixed with various herbs that haven't proven to do anything good for you and will probably damage your health. Plus, they are a huge rip-off since they don't cost much to make but they cost a lot of money to buy.

These pills and capsules will undoubtedly put needless strain on not only your heart but also your Endocrine and Nervous System--not to mention the strain on your wallet. Use the money you save to buy wild salmon! This is definitely not good for you; your body works hard to restore these systems while you're sleeping and when you work out by flushing them free of bodily contaminants. These artificial stimulants add undue stress to your body's repair mechanisms and will most probably lead to:

- Exhaustion
- Central Nervous System Burnout
- Aggressiveness and Mood swings
- Mental Fatigue
- Psychological problems (depression, anxiety etc.)
- Hamper your body's ability to recover from everyday stress

It's just not worth it for all these reasons. Furthermore, they don't really work. When it comes down to it, losing fat is about two things: Proper Nutrition and Exercise. If you're eating healthy foods when you're hungry (see the recommended food lists above) and you are doing a healthy level of cardio and strength training each week you will lose weight. You should be re-learning how to lead a better, healthier lifestyle because that's where you have failed before by falling for "quick fixes." You must retrain your brain and by the end of that you will have it all come together!

The only thing that these *'Fat Burners'* advertise that is true is that they contain caffeine. Now, caffeine does help you melt off fat in a variety of ways including managing blood sugar levels and allowing the metabolism and consumption of stored fat. Caffeine is also useful as a pre-workout stimulant and it's pretty good at this. It will give you mental clearness and allows you to work fiercer. But using natural stimulants that won't cost you a ton of money contain enough caffeine to be damaging to you so be cautious.

**Coffee**

Black coffee is good. Have an Americano or down a shot of Espresso before your workout. This is the most pure and most trustworthy form of caffeine available and it's natural and cheap. A little bag of coffee only costs you a small portion of what a bottle of Fat Burners will and will save your health--you'll get the same results anyway!

**Yerba Mate**

This is a long-established tea from South America. It is highly trendy in places like Argentina and Brazil. It warms up your body and helps to activate your body's fat burning metabolic processes. It also has a more soothing stimulating effect than coffee so it's a great substitute for people who don't fare too well with caffeine from coffee. It's also cheap and can is available at most health stores. Buy the "loose" type and make a strong brew. It contains a lot of anti-oxidants and also provides you with minerals which is a big plus to its detoxing and fat burning abilities.

**Green Tea**

Surely, all of you have heard about green tea. The hype is true. This substance truly is a great energizer and refresher for the our bodies; it has been proven to:

- Help Burn Fat
- Raise Metabolism
- Relax the Mind and Body
- Be a Potent Anti-Oxidant
- Anti-Estrogenic

Again ensure you buy the loose variety. It's cheaper and fresher. A few glasses a day is recommended as the best option for people whose bodies don't do well with any caffeine from whatever source.

**Chapter 16: Relax Your Way to Fierce Abs**

There are actual physiological changes that happen to your body when under stress that can cause you to stack on more pounds than when you aren't stressed. These changes are triggered in our *adrenal glands*, which control the stress response and many other basic bodily functions. When your adrenals not in balance, your body prepares for adversity the best way it knows how: It stores calories. If we re-establish our adrenal glands back to normal, healthy function, cravings go away, energy levels go back up and obstinate pounds burn away easier.

We usually think that "being stressed-out" is an emotional state, but the body thinks of stress as a physical state. One of the ways it physically handles stress is by being sparing with how it makes use of calories, storing them mainly as fat in the abdominal area.

The way we evolved this way has a lot to do with living in the wild. If you were being chased by a wild animal, your adrenals shifted immediately into fight-or-flight mode: They release adrenaline and cortisol into your blood and these chemicals help to give us a large boost of strength and rapidly activated energy creation from carbohydrates and fats. Once the threat was gone, our instincts made us replenish with calorie-dense foods. These foods are most easily stored as fat. Under the influence of cortisol, we are less sensitive to leptin; leptin is the hormone that signals our body that we are full, so with low leptin sensitivity we will eat more than we need to be satisfied. Not good for weight loss at all...

Stress can be reduced by simple methods, some of which are what this book is all about: Eating healthy and regularly and getting a lot of exercise. Just doing this will help you de-stress. Also, getting proper sleep matters. Sleeping proper hours lets your muscles grow and de-stresses you (hence my article http://bit.ly/14i2dbb).

De-stress yourself during the day as well. Here are two easy and fun ways to do that:

**Breathe.** Three to four deep breaths (breathe through your nose) can slow your heart rate and calm your whole body. Make time throughout the day to just breathe, especially when you feel stressed. It doesn't take long to breathe deeply a few times. Learn to be acquainted with the signals your body and brain send you that you need to take a break. Breathe, get some fresh air, have a cup of herbal tea, and put your feet up for a while. It doesn't take long to do this.

**Play.** Even as an adult, make having fun a priority! Many of us forget that just a few minutes of fun or a good laugh can be very relaxing. I'm giving you a virtual prescription: "Play!"

## Chapter 17: Final Tips and Summary

1.) WEIGHTS- I'm sure many of you have grabbed a 20 lb. plate or dumbbell and crunched to your side. Or have done weighted rope crunches; but are you doing too much? Weighted ab exercises are great for getting that "ripped look" or "popped" look you often see on many cover models but using too much can ruin your physique. Doing too many weighted ab exercises may actually ADD inches to your waist. If you like to add weights like me, train abs with weights no more than 3-4 sets and only 2-3 times a week with a rep range of around 12-15.

2.) LOWER ABS- lower abs are the hardest part of the core to build because the body (especially in men) stores a lot of fat in the lower abdomen. I get tons of questions about this one particular area! Most of you are doing lower abdominal exercises wrong! And fitness magazines are not always telling you the right way either. To fully work your lower abs correctly try the roman chair leg raises, or lying leg raises. The key is to bring your feet entirely up to your head and/ or chest, otherwise you're not working much other than your hip flexors (hips basically).

3.) OBLIQUES- If you want to get that glorious V going on with your obliques like me then you need to twist. Try doing weighted medicine ball twists or broomstick twists--but here's the trick: Don't use your arms to move the ball. Keep them rigid and use your obliques! I do these on a decline bench with a weight or ball and also on the bosu ball.

4.) DURATION- If you hit your abs hard then you should be in pain in about 20 minutes. Mix up the rest periods using no more than 1 minute breaks and keep changing your routine by changing up the rest times.

5.) WEEKLY- Because we use our abs every single day in all that we do we can train them every day as well. It doesn't take much to sculpt and/or build than if you hit them hard and make them burn. Every other day will put you in the 3-4 times per week range.

6.) REPS- I'm going to repeat, doing 1,000 crunches at a time won't get you abs. What will? Controlling your movement and not using any type of momentum to propel you forward. Your abs should be doing the work, not the momentum! Also, if you're not feeling your abs being worked then change it up! There is always something to do to make it harder.

7.) WE ALL HAVE ABS- Did you know most bodybuilders don't exercise their abs specifically (maybe 100 crunches once a week but that's all). Your thinking I'm insane right now I'm sure…But its true and the reason is simple! Once you decrease your body fat percentage, your abs will reveal themselves. Working abs is more about sculpting them. Drop your body fat percent by eating continuously the right foods and train your body right and I guarantee you will see those bad boys!

I want you to know that you have a real shot at achieving those Fierce Abs you have always wanted! And keep in mind that everyone's definition of *Fierce* is different. Some want a ripped six pack and others just want a tighter mid-section. Whatever your goal is I am here to help you and I truly hope that this book and the accompanying Fierce Abs workout series will help and motivate you to take action. I want to see you succeed and reach your goals. I wish you the best of luck and look forward to what lies ahead.

## Questions or Comments?

I'd love to hear from you. You can email me at jess@fierceabs.com.

**Need Help?**

I routinely help clients train, prepare for events, develop nutrition regimens, recover from an accident, and more. You can reach me at jess@fierceabs.com to get more information on any of the products or services that I offer.

**One Last Thing...**

If you feel that you have gained something personally as a result of reading this book or the free video series it would mean the world to me if you would take a few minutes and post your review directly on Amazon. Just click here (http://amzn.to/Z4UOJk) and it will take you directly to the page:

Your Friend and Trainer,

Jess

Made in the USA
Lexington, KY
06 October 2013